Core Competencies for Psychiatric Education

Defining, Teaching, and Assessing
Resident Competence

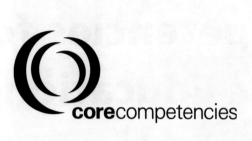

Core Competencies for Psychiatric Education

Defining, Teaching, and Assessing Resident Competence

Linda Boerger Andrews, M.D.
Director of Residency Education, General Psychiatry Residency Program
Assistant Dean, Office of Student Affairs
Baylor College of Medicine, Houston, Texas

John William Burruss, M.D.
Associate Director of Residency Education, General Psychiatry Residency Program
Chief of Psychiatry, Ben Taub General Hospital
Baylor College of Medicine, Houston, Texas

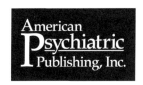

American Psychiatric Publishing, Inc.

Washington, DC
London, England

Copyright © 2004 American Psychiatric Publishing, Inc.
ALL RIGHTS RESERVED

Manufactured in the United States of America on acid-free paper
08 07 06 05 04   5 4 3 2 1
First Edition

Typeset in Adobe's Berling Roman and Frutiger 55 Roman

American Psychiatric Publishing, Inc.
1000 Wilson Boulevard
Arlington, VA 22209-3901
www.appi.org

Library of Congress Cataloging-in-Publication Data
Andrews, Linda Boerger, 1963–
    Core competencies for psychiatric education : defining, teaching, and assessing resident competence / Linda Boerger Andrews, John William Burruss.
        p. ; cm.
    Includes bibliographical references and index.
    ISBN 1-58562-130-7 (alk. paper)
    1. Psychiatry—Study and teaching (Residency)—United States. 2. Psychotherapy—Study and teaching—United States.
3. Core competencies—United States. 4. Clinical competence—Standards. I. Burruss, John William, 1966– II. Title.
    [DNLM: 1. Internship and Residency—standards. 2. Psychiatry—education. 3. Clinical Competence—standards.
4. Competency-Based Education—methods. WM 19.5 A567c 2004]
RC459.5.U6A537 2004
616.89′0071′173—dc22

2003063564

British Library Cataloguing in Publication Data
A CIP record is available from the British Library.

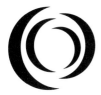

Contents

Appendixes

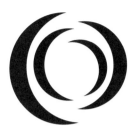

Part I

Introduction to the Competencies

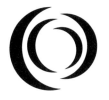

Introduction to Program Accreditation and Board Certification

Every person actively involved with psychiatric residency education should have some understanding of the accreditation process for training programs and the mechanism for board certification of independent practitioners. This requires at least a basic knowledge of the Psychiatry Residency Review Committee (RRC) of the Accreditation Council for Graduate Medical Education (ACGME) and the American Board of Psychiatry and Neurology (ABPN), one of the member organizations of the American Board of Medical Specialties (ABMS). In short, the ACGME, through its Psychiatry RRC, is responsible for maintaining the accreditation of psychiatry training *programs*, while the ABPN's mission is "promoting excellence in the practice of psychiatry" by *individual practitioners* (www.abpn.com). These two unique functions are inextricably related, as will be detailed in this chapter.

The ACGME is the private accreditation organization for residency education programs in the United States. As an organization, the ACGME is composed of 26 individual RRCs that provide guidelines for each of 110 different specialties and subspecialties. Additionally, the ACGME provides guidelines for the institutions that sponsor graduate medical education programs. Note that these two accreditations, program and institution, are separate and distinct from each other, but they are equally necessary for an institution to continue to host residency training programs. Loss of ac-

creditation for a given program ends the institution's participation in graduate medical education in that particular specialty and any associated subspecialties. Loss of institutional accreditation jeopardizes all residency training in every specialty and subspecialty occurring within that institution.

To create the guidelines that detail minimum required elements of a residency program, or "program requirements" as they are commonly known, the individual RRCs solicit the input of various interested parties, or "stakeholders," as detailed on the ACGME website (www.acgme.org). The stakeholders include physicians in the specialty, training directors, trainees, sponsoring institutions, governmental entities, and the general public. The program requirements explicitly define the minimum necessary clinical rotations, supervision, didactic educational components, and other mandatory aspects of a residency training experience. To ensure that programs are implementing the requirements appropriately, the RRC sends site visitors to review each program on a regular basis. The site visitors may be generalists, with broad experience in education, or specialists who are experienced in residency education in the specialty of the program being reviewed. Site visits occur at any interval from 1 to 5 years, with the longer intervals reserved for programs with an established track record for consistent quality and compliance with the educational program requirements.

In September 1997, the ACGME shifted its emphasis from assessing a program's *potential* to educate residents (as determined by compliance with the structure and timing elements of the program requirements) to determining each program's actual success in educating residents (Leach 2001). Success will be measured by evaluating the desired *outcome* of trainees' achieved competence in six specific areas. In other words, did the program in fact reach its potential in educating residents? It is this shift in emphasis, and the subsequent need of residency training directors and residency programs to demonstrate compliance with the new expectations of the ACGME, that provide the impetus for this manual.

This philosophical change within the ACGME had its origin in the Robert Wood Johnson Foundation–funded Outcome Project. Substantial investigation into other areas of healthcare, business, and education resulted in the realization that the accreditation methods used in residency training had become anachronistic. Legislatures, accrediting bodies, state boards of education, and internal reviewers all want to know if the education of students is having the desired effect (Morreale and Backlund 1999). The use of timed requirements and exposure to certain minimum amounts of clinical and didactic material was no longer felt to be sufficient to attest to the *ability* of physicians to practice their craft, though the program requirements were still thought to be markers for a program's potential to educate competent physicians. The Outcome Project was therefore born, with the guiding principles that 1) whatever we measure we improve, 2) programs need more flexibility to be creative, and 3) public accountability must be served (Leach 2001). Major changes in the accreditation process for residency education have resulted from the Outcome Project such that training directors will now be charged with

- Ensuring that the program provides the ACGME-defined elements of an adequate curriculum with attention to including all six of the core competencies.
- Establishing goals and objectives for each step in the training process that incorporate the necessary milestones toward achieved competence in the six areas.
- Devising and implementing evaluation instruments that accurately assess attained competence in all six competencies.
- Testing for progress toward competence by each trainee.
- Measuring that progress for each individual trainee and for the program as a whole.

- Reviewing the curriculum based on the collected outcome data of trainees' competence.
- Modifying the training experience over time to correct any areas of deficiency.

It should be remembered that the term *outcomes*, as used in this book, refers to educational outcomes rather than clinical outcomes. The end result of clinical care, whether a favorable or untoward event for a given patient or set of patients, may be used to help determine competency, but this usage of the term should not be confused with an educational outcome. *Educational outcomes* refers to trainees' learning and incorporating a set of prescribed knowledge and skills into their practice of medicine, regardless of the outcome for any individual patient. It follows that a resident may provide thoroughly competent care in every way, and yet this may still be followed by an adverse clinical outcome. The theory behind the ACGME's change to emphasizing the achievement of competencies (an educational outcome) is that the probability of unfortunate clinical outcomes will be diminished when accredited programs train physicians to employ competent care.

The General Competencies requirements that have resulted from the Outcome Project are currently being phased in for all core residency training programs in the United States. As of July 2002, programs that are not felt to be making adequate efforts to achieve compliance with the new requirements will be subject to citation from the ACGME site reviewers. Recognizing the tremendous complexity and labor involved in making this dramatic philosophical shift, the ACGME has expressed its full support for sharing successes from programs that are making rapid progress toward implementing measures of competency so that all programs do not have to create entire measuring systems and evaluation methods independently. Information will be disseminated to residency program directors as these successful programs are identified. Information can be found on the ACGME website, in residency program directors' forums (including computer-based formats, via listserves and chat rooms, and within other association-based communication) at various educational meetings, and within the various RRC newsletters.

The Psychiatry RRC is headed administratively by a full-time executive director. As of this writing, the executive director position is held by Larry Sultan, Ph.D. Joel Silverman, M.D., is the chair of the Psychiatry RRC itself, which comprises 18 experienced and dedicated educators. The Psychiatry RRC is charged with maintaining and ensuring the standards for breadth and quality in general psychiatric residency education in this country, as well as for the five psychiatry subspecialty training areas: Child and Adolescent Psychiatry, Addiction Psychiatry, Forensic Psychiatry, Geriatric Psychiatry, and Pain Management Psychiatry. It is expected that there will soon be a sixth accredited specialty representing the consultation-liaison psychiatry field, called Psychosomatic Psychiatry. Contact information for the RRC is available on the ACGME website in the Residency Review Committee section. The Psychiatry RRC has added requirements for five specific Psychotherapy Competencies in addition to the six General Competencies of the ACGME. Chapter 2 of this book is dedicated to outlining the six General Competencies and the five Psychotherapy Competencies.

The ABMS works closely with the ACGME. As stated previously, whereas the ACGME and its associated RRCs are concerned with accrediting the residency training programs in this country, the various specialty boards are concerned with certifying the individual practitioners within any given specialty. The two agencies are functionally inseparable, however, as admissibility to sit for board examination (note that the ABMS specialty boards do not use the term *board eligible*) requires successful completion of an ACGME-approved residency program. Likewise, one component of ongoing ACGME accreditation for residency training programs is acceptable passage rates of specialty board examinations by the graduates of the residency training program.

Whereas the ACGME is composed of 26 RRCs, the ABMS incorporates 24 medical specialty boards and provides coordination of their activities while disseminating information to the many interested parties in the United States. The stated mission of this organization, according to its website (www.abms.org), is "to maintain and improve the quality of medical care in the United States." It also maintains and distributes a current listing of all "diplomates," or board-certified physicians, in all ABMS member specialties.

As mentioned previously, the member board for psychiatry is the American Board of Psychiatry and Neurology, or ABPN. Founded in 1934, the ABPN is a nonprofit corporation with a mission to "serve the public interest by promoting excellence in the practice of psychiatry and neurology through lifelong certification including competency testing processes" (www.abpn.com). The ABPN is made up of 16 members that are elected to their positions. The members come from the American Psychiatric Association (APA), American Medical Association (AMA), American Neurological Association, and American Academy of Neurology, with equal distribution of members from psychiatry and neurology. An executive vice president provides administrative management of the board. Stephen C. Scheiber, M.D., has provided this leadership for many years.

In parallel to the process of the ACGME, the ABMS, under the leadership of David Leach, M.D., created a Task Force on Competence. This group recommended adoption of the same six competencies into the member boards' work with certification and recertification. This recommendation has now been accepted by the ABMS and is being implemented. Here again, the accrediting bodies for both residency training programs and individual practitioners have sustained their separate but inextricable relationship. Additionally, this step by the ABMS has taken the competencies from the realm of residency education into the broader world of lifelong learning. Every practitioner who will be certified or recertified over time will need to develop some sophistication with the competency concept and will need to ensure his or her self-education in these areas.

Dr. Stephen C. Scheiber, Dr. Thomas A. M. Kramer, and Susan E. Adamowski, the executive leadership of the ABPN, have recently published a book on the competencies from the ABPN's perspective. This volume, entitled *Core Competencies for Psychiatric Practice: What Clinicians Need to Know* (Scheiber et al. 2003), is a must read for anyone facing certification or recertification with the ABPN.

References

Leach DC: The ACGME Competencies: substance or form. J Am Coll Surg 192(3):396–398, 2001

Morreale SP, Backlund PA: Assessment: Coming of Age. Washington, DC, National Communication Association, 1999. Available at: http://www.natcom.org/Instruction/assessment/Assessment/article99.htm. Accessed January 28, 2003.

Scheiber SC, Kramer TAM, Adamowski SE: Core Competencies for Psychiatric Practice: What Clinicians Need to Know (A Report of the American Board of Psychiatry and Neurology, Inc). Washington, DC, American Psychiatric Publishing, 2003

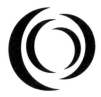

2

ACGME General Competencies and Psychiatry RRC Psychotherapy Competencies

At its February 1999 meeting, the Accreditation Council for Graduate Medical Education (ACGME) endorsed competencies for residents in six general areas: patient care, medical knowledge, practice-based learning and improvement, interpersonal and communication skills, professionalism, and systems-based practice (www.acgme.org). The general competencies were identified by means of a thorough and collaborative review process occurring between January 1998 and February 1999. The extensive input and feedback process involved published reports, curriculum documents, surveys, interviews, and focus groups. It tapped a cross section of key stakeholders with representation from the medical profession, residents and educators, employers of physicians, patients, and society at large as typified by private foundations, the U.S. government, healthcare quality monitors, and community health providers. Executives representing nursing, physician assistants, and allied health professionals were also involved. The Outcome Project Advisory Group reviewed a compilation of the data and made the "cut" from an original list of 86 statements to the present six General Competencies (www.acgme.org/outcome/about/faq.asp).

Identification of the General Competencies was the first step in a long-term effort designed to emphasize educational outcome assessment in residency programs and in the accreditation process. By identifying the General Competencies, the ACGME was responding in part to a growing criticism from a variety of sources, including the medical community itself, that residents were not adequately prepared to practice in the rapidly changing healthcare environment. From an educational standpoint, competencies can be regarded as the logical building blocks on which assessments of professional development are based. In the case of graduate medical education, identification of the General Competencies represents specification of what residents should know and be able to do. When competencies are identified, a program can effectively determine the objectives that should guide progress toward their achievement and, in turn, what outcomes should be assessed as evidence of the program's quality (i.e., its effectiveness in meeting the objectives and thus preparing competent residents for practice) (www.acgme.org).

Most accrediting bodies in the health professions, education, and business have focused on educational outcomes since the 1980s. At that time, the U.S. Department of Education mandated a movement aimed at making greater use of outcome assessment in accreditation. As a result, efforts were begun by these organizations to expand their use of outcome measures in accreditation. In addition, since the U.S. system of medical education depends heavily on public funding, medical educators are called on to offer evidence of their responsible stewardship in preparing competent physicians to meet the healthcare needs of the public that supports their efforts. The ability to demonstrate educational outcomes as the achievement of competency-based learning objectives provides just such evidence (www.acgme.org).

The Outcome Project refers to *educational* outcomes (not to be confused with clinical outcomes; see Chapter 1) as "evidence showing the degree to which program purposes and objectives are or are not being attained, including achievement of appropriate skills and competencies by students" (www.acgme.org/outcome/comp/compFull.asp). Clinical outcomes can and should be used as educational outcomes for several of the General Competencies. However, they are not the only educational outcomes for residency education. Achievement of learning is the ultimate purpose of any well-structured educational activity. In keeping with the ACGME's mission to ensure and improve the quality of graduate medical education, the Outcome Project focuses on educational outcomes, thus demonstrating achievement of learning by graduates of the accredited residency education programs. At present, graduate medical education accreditation utilizes a "minimum threshold model" by which programs are judged according to how they comply with minimum standards established by the Residency Review Committees (RRCs) and the ACGME. In the competency-based model toward which the Outcome Project is directed, programs will be asked to show how residents have achieved competency-based educational objectives and, in turn, how programs use information drawn from evaluation of those objectives to improve the educational experience of the residents. Stated another way, the minimum threshold model identifies whether a program has the potential to educate residents; the competency-based model examines whether the program is actually educating them.

Since 1999, the ACGME's RRCs and Institutional Review Committees have incorporated the General Competencies into their requirements. Most program requirements now specify that the residency program must require its residents to develop the competencies in the six areas to the level expected of a new practitioner. Toward this end, programs must define the specific knowledge, skills, and attitudes required and provide educational experiences as needed in order for their residents to demonstrate the competencies. Without exception, all program requirements now include reference to the need for goals and objectives as well as evaluation of the residents and the program. Many program requirements also already include references to the General Competencies, although the language may vary somewhat from the minimum language approved by the ACGME in

September 1999. The critical step is linking assessment with specific learning objectives. Programs must evaluate whether or not they are completing this important assessment-linking step and, if they are, whether they are using the results of their evaluations to improve their program.

A brief description of the six General Competencies, as currently endorsed by the ACGME, follows. A list of the ACGME's recommended specific knowledge, skills, and attitudes to be assessed within each of the six general competencies can be found in Chapter 5 of this book.

ACGME General Competencies

Patient Care

The ACGME Outcome Project description of this competency states that residents must be able to provide patient care that is compassionate, appropriate, and effective for the treatment of health problems and the promotion of health. This competency focuses on patient management. Competent residents will be expected to use algorithms, practice guidelines, and a synthesis of available data to determine how to treat patients' health problems and to promote their overall health.

Medical Knowledge

The ACGME Outcome Project description of this competency states that residents must demonstrate knowledge about established and evolving biomedical, clinical, and cognate (epidemiological and social-behavioral) sciences and application of this knowledge to patient care. This competency focuses on the residents' knowledge of current scientific information, clinical trials, and new developments, advances, and treatment options for patients. This competency emphasizes more the *what* and *why* aspects of medicine rather than the *how*, which is better captured by the patient care competency.

Practice-Based Learning and Improvement

The ACGME Outcome Project description of this competency states that residents must be able to investigate and evaluate their patient care practices, appraise and assimilate scientific evidence, and improve their patient care practices. This competency focuses on a resident's ability to identify errors or gaps that may be reflected by national, regional, or local practice data. Residents should demonstrate an ability to determine how these shortfalls might be addressed.

Interpersonal and Communication Skills

The ACGME Outcome Project description of this competency states that residents must be able to demonstrate interpersonal and communication skills that result in effective information exchange and teaming with patients, their patients' families, and professional associates.

Professionalism

The ACGME Outcome Project description of this competency states that residents must demonstrate a commitment to carrying out professional responsibilities, adherence to ethical principles, and sensitivity to a diverse patient population. This competency will include content emphasizing confidentiality, informed consent, privacy, and withholding of clinical care. This competency covers areas of physician responsibility and ethics.

Systems-Based Practice

The ACGME Outcome Project description for this competency states that residents must demonstrate an awareness of and responsiveness to the larger context and system of health care and the ability to effectively draw on system resources to provide care that is of optimal value. This competency emphasizes issues or content dealing with professional practice within the larger system, such as state or federal agencies and the regulations they issue, advocacy for quality patient care, assistance for patients within the larger system, and insurance. Systems-based care is generally thought not to represent a multidisciplinary team within a hospital, clinic, or other organization.

The Program Requirements for Residency Training in Psychiatry and Residency Education in Child and Adolescent Psychiatry, Addiction Psychiatry, Forensic Psychiatry, and Geriatric Psychiatry include specific language on the six General Competencies under the Internal Evaluation section (www.acgme.org/RRC_ progReq/ 400pr101.pdf). The Program Requirements for Residency Education in Pain Management (Psychiatry) do not include specific language about the six General Competencies. These program requirements became effective in 2000, and it is expected that they will incorporate General Competency language into their next revision.

The Program Requirements for Residency Training in Psychiatry state in section VI.B ("Evaluation of Resident Competencies") the following (www.acgme.org/ RRC_progReq/400pr101.pdf):

The residency program must demonstrate that it has an effective plan for assessing resident performance throughout the program and for utilizing assessment results to improve resident performance.

1. This plan should include use of dependable measures to assess residents' competence in

    a. patient care
    b. medical knowledge
    c. practice-based learning and improvement
    d. interpersonal and communication skills
    e. professionalism, and
    f. systems-based practice

2. A mechanism must be in place for providing regular and timely performance feedback to residents which utilizes assessment results to achieve progressive improvements in the performance of residents in each competency area.

3. Programs that do not have a set of measures in place must develop a plan for improving their evaluations or demonstrate progress in implementing such a plan.

4. The program must provide documented evidence to demonstrate that the proficiency/ competence of each resident is assessed using techniques that may include supervisory reports, videotapes, oral examinations, case reports, patient care observations, or other methods.

The Program Requirements also weave many of the six General Competencies into the body of the text in sections V: "The Educational Program" (A. "Objectives of Training"; B. "Curriculum"; and D. "Other Required Components") and VI: "Internal Evaluation" (A. "Evaluation of Residents"; B. "Evaluation of Resident Competencies"; and C. "Program Evaluation") (www.acgme.org/ RRC_progReq/400pr101.pdf).

The Program Requirements for Residency Education in Child and Adolescent Psychiatry state in section VII.A ("Evaluation of Residents") (see www.acgme.org/RRC_ progReq/400pr101.pdf):

Programs must develop at least one written core competency for its residents in each of the following areas:

    a. clinical science
    b. interpersonal skills and communication
    c. patient care
    d. practice-based learning and improvement
    e. professionalism and ethical behavior
    f. systems-based practice

The program must provide documented evidence to demonstrate that the proficiency/competence of each resident is assessed using techniques that may include supervisory reports, videotapes, oral examinations, case reports, patient care observations, or other methods.

Both the American Association of Directors of Psychiatric Residency Training (AADPRT) and the Association for Academic Psychiatry (AAP) have developed task forces and work groups to address defining, implementing, and assessing the six General Competencies. Both are currently using their respective websites (www. aadprt. org and www.academicpsychiatry.org) to serve as clearinghouses for ideas and ongoing discussions about the six General Competencies. Similarly, the Work Group on Training and Education of the American Academy of Child and Adolescent Psychiatry has developed sample written core competencies for each area. These samples are meant to serve as potential models for program directors as they develop ways to implement the competencies (Sexson et al. 2001).

Since January 2001, the Program Requirements for Residency Training in Psychiatry have included specific Psychotherapy Competencies in addition to the General Competencies. The Program Requirements text delineates the Psychotherapy Competencies in section VI.B ("Evaluation of Resident Competencies") as follows (www.acgme.org/RRC_progReq/400pr101.pdf):

> The program must demonstrate that residents have achieved competency in at least the following forms of treatment:

> a. brief therapy
> b. cognitive-behavioral therapy
> c. combined psychotherapy and psychopharmacology
> d. psychodynamic therapy, and
> e. supportive therapy

Every residency program director should review the Program Requirements to ensure the program has a clear understanding of what the RRC expects regarding the five Psychotherapy Competencies. The Task Force on Competency of the AADPRT developed sample competencies for each of the five Psychotherapy Competencies. The work groups who helped the task force develop the competencies were made up of residency training directors, psychotherapy experts from within AADPRT, representatives from the American Psychiatric Association's Commission on Psychotherapy, and resident representatives. These sample competencies have each undergone several revisions based on feedback from all work group and task force members. The sample competencies are available on the AADPRT website (www.aadprt.org) and are included in Chapter 6 of this book.

References

Sexson S, Sargent J, Zima B, et al: Sample core competencies in child and adolescent psychiatry training: a starting point. Acad Psychiatry 25(4):201–213, 2001

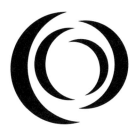

Part II

Teaching and Assessing the Competencies

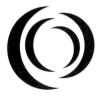

3

How Residents Learn and Develop Competence

Skill acquisition is a developmental process. Competence is developed over time and is nurtured by reflection on experience. A model of knowledge and skill acquisition that is simple and relevant for medicine has been developed by Hubert and Stuart Dreyfus (see Epstein and Hundert 2002; Leach 2002). The named stages of novice, advanced beginner, competent, proficient, expert, and master expand our understanding of competence and offer alternatives that reflect the developmental nature of competence. For each of the six General Competencies, there are rules that must be learned (novice, advanced beginner) and these rules must be applied in increasingly complex contexts (competent, proficient, expert, master). Ideally, medical students progress from novice to advanced beginners, and residents from advanced beginners to competent. Residency education should systematically foster development from advanced beginner to competent. To be competent, residents must be involved enough to be accountable. So, in this model of competency development, moving from advanced beginner to competent means less detachment and greater immersion in particular contexts.

This model, described in Leach's editorial in *JAMA* (Leach 2002), characterizes the progress as moving from rule-based behaviors to context-based behaviors. As residents encounter particular patients and attempt to apply the correct rules, they are forced to select a perspective and assign relevance to multiple pieces of information. Not all the details of a particular case are of equal importance; some are more relevant than others in a given case. Learners select which details are more rel-

evant and in doing so, select a perspective from which to view the case. At this stage (competent), the result depends on the perspective adopted by the learner.

When mistakes are made, learners usually make one of two responses: 1) detach and create new rules to prevent future similar mistakes or 2) investigate in a reflective manner how the mistakes occurred. The latter response eventually leads to and reinforces accurate pattern recognition. For example, it is not uncommon for good clinicians to recognize a disease within a few minutes and then to spend the next few minutes confirming or denying that initial impression. Rules become subliminal and integrated with intuition. Tacit knowledge (knowledge that is accurate but hard to explain) emerges. Tacit knowledge is practically automatic or equivalent to a habit. It is knowledge that is difficult to articulate or identify directly. "You know it when you see it" (Epstein and Hundert 2002; Leach 2002). A medical student interviews a patient for 2 hours and writes 10 pages of history and physical examination to describe the patient and discuss a differential diagnosis. A resident interviews the same patient for 30 minutes and writes a one-page summary that includes all of the pertinent positive and negative findings and a thorough, but brief, discussion of the differential diagnosis. A senior faculty member interviews the same patient for 15 minutes at the bedside and then presents a case summary, including all pertinent findings and the most likely diagnosis. Rules have given way to tacit knowledge, habits of pattern recognition informed by previous mistakes and applied to a new patient situation.

Residents acquire competence in this fashion. They, first, obtain factual knowledge and then develop skills by practicing through experience. They develop integrative abilities by adapting their initially obtained skills to new situations. They learn to manage ambiguous problems and to tolerate uncertainty. Eventually, they develop the ability to make decisions even with limited information. Proceeding to this final stage requires repeated action, followed by assessment, especially of mistakes, and then modification of action. It also requires developing the ability to draw on several strategies for solving problems and not just using the same strategy to solve all problems, which is how most novices approach problem-solving tasks.

Expert clinicians often use pattern recognition for routine problems and hypothetico-deductive reasoning for complex problems outside their area of expertise (Epstein and Hundert 2002). Ideally, residents are given the opportunity to evaluate and treat a large enough number of patients so that they can develop pattern recognition. They must also be challenged to evaluate and treat patients, with adequate supervision, in unfamiliar settings, with new diagnostic questions, with ambiguous problems, and with limited information available to them. They should be given opportunities (clinical and didactic) to learn firsthand what is relatively common, from a diagnostic and treatment perspective. They, then, should be asked to stretch their basic knowledge and skills to apply them to patients with less common diagnostic problems or with treatment strategies for treatment-resistant patients.

Residents should be exposed to multiple approaches to patient assessment, diagnosis, and treatment planning. This should occur through supervisory contact with many clinicians, in as many different clinical settings as possible, seeing patients across the disease severity continuum and from more to less common psychiatric illnesses and illness presentations. Learning theory suggests that multiple learning trials and teaching methods (repetition), specific and timely feedback, and ownership of one's actions all contribute positively to overall learning effectiveness and "habit development."

Since competence is developmental, a comprehensive view of competence implies that multiple types of assessment are conducted over time to discern development. Assessment must take into account what is assessed, how it is assessed, and the assessment's usefulness in fostering future learning. Good assessment is a form of learning and should provide guidance and support to address learning needs. Within each knowledge, skill, and attitude domain, there are four levels at which

a trainee might be assessed (Miller 1990). The *knows* level refers to the recall of facts, principles, and theories. The *knows how* level involves the ability to solve problems and describe procedures. The *shows how* level usually involves human (standardized patients), mechanical, or computer simulations that involve demonstration of skills in a controlled setting. The *does* level refers to observations of real practice. For each of these levels, the student can demonstrate the ability to imitate or replicate a protocol, apply principles in a familiar situation, adapt principles to new situations, and associate new knowledge with previously learned principles (Epstein and Hundert 2002). These four levels provide a framework within which to think about resident learning and one to be used when selecting evaluation tools to best match the assessment of the six General Competencies and the five Psychotherapy Competencies.

Residents' performance in real practice would be the most preferred way to assess knowledge, skills, and attitude mastery and competence. Subjective clinical evaluations and individual supervision probably provide the most effective means for assessing the *does* level of knowledge, skills, and attitudes for most of the six General Competencies and the five Psychotherapy Competencies. This would be especially true if multiple evaluations by multiple people following repeated direct observation of residents' work were completed. In fact, Whitcomb (2002) suggested that the only way to determine that a resident is competent is to critically observe the resident caring for patients in a variety of clinical settings and under different clinical circumstances. He argues that what is needed to improve graduate medical education and competency assessment is not new methods of assessment of residents but a better system for documenting the faculty's observations of residents' daily work in clinical settings.

The final comment about learning is really more about systems than about individuals. Individual learning will be most effective when it occurs within a system that encourages learner self-assessment, peer review and accountability, and lifelong learning, in which teachers continue to view themselves as learners. For example, systems that demonstrate that individual assessment data (assessment of individual residents) can lead to systemic changes and improvements (changes in residency program curricula) will motivate more meaningful feedback and evaluation exchanges. In turn, hopefully, better teaching will occur, individuals will be able to develop greater competence, and the larger system will become accustomed to a state of continuous quality improvement (Epstein and Hundert 2002).

References

Epstein R, Hundert M: Defining and assessing professional competence. JAMA 287(2):226–235, 2002

Leach D: Competence is a habit (editorial). JAMA 287(2): 243–244, 2002

Miller G: The assessment of clinical skills/competence/performance. Acad Med 65(suppl):63–67, 1990

Whitcomb M: Competency-based graduate medical education? Of course! But how should competency be assessed? Acad Med 77:359–360, 2002

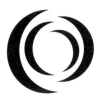

4

How to Assess Learning and Competence

Defining the Goals of Assessment

The act of overtly measuring various aspects of performance will foster trainees' greater awareness and incorporation of the skills being measured. Put a different way, "You get what you measure" (Hensinger 2001). It is therefore crucial that the residency program director and residency program curriculum committee carefully decide on the variables to be measured early in the process of implementing the competencies. Failure to do so could result in a program measuring behaviors that are not paramount to competent physician behavior, leading to problematic situations. The process of carefully selecting the goals of assessment will ensure that as learners "learn to the test" and teachers "teach to the test," the test is actually measuring those qualities that are desirable to be measured. Likewise, the qualities most desirable in trainees will be accentuated and learners will focus on the skills that educators want them to develop. "The test" in this case consists of the many evaluations completed over the course of a given trainee's career in a residency program. The items chosen for evaluation should be communicated fully to the learners from the very beginning of their training and reemphasized with each feedback session, final rotation evaluation, and semiannual residency training director's evaluation.

The overarching goal throughout a program's assessment scheme will be, of necessity, establishing the program's success at creating competent residents in the six General Competencies and five specific Psychotherapy Competencies outlined extensively in this book. Residency programs will vary widely in the manner of measuring these attributes and in the process of defining success at achieving trainee competence. This will lead to varied educational goals within different residency programs, and a set of "best practices" will emerge over time. A detailed "to-do list" to be used in establishing these educational goals within a psychiatric residency training program can be found in Chapter 8.

Defining the specific components to be measured within each general area of competency is an important part of each residency program's effort to achieve compliance with the ACGME requirements. Chapter 6 devotes a significant amount of attention to the many different aspects of each general area of competency, though the exact nature and quantifiability of each competency aspect remain uncertain.

Distinguishing Feedback From Evaluation

It is tremendously important for all teaching physicians to make the distinction between *feedback* and *evaluation*. The differences between these two forms of teacher-learner interaction are surprisingly difficult to master and require almost continual practice to implement effectively. Perhaps the most important difference between the two, and a meaningful way to distinguish one from the other, lies in the *formative* nature of feedback when compared with the *summative* nature of evaluation. The *American Heritage Dictionary* (2nd Col-

Table 1. Differences between feedback and evaluation

	Feedback	Evaluation
Intention	Shapes and improves future behavior by accentuating strengths and establishing areas in which improvement is needed	Comments on behavior that has already occurred and serves as a final judgment and assessment of the quality of that behavior
Format	Usually verbal	Usually written
Scope	Small, specific, discrete portions	Comprehensive and more general approach
Language	Neutral statements of fact	Language that defines the value and quality of a performance compared with a norm
	Avoids evaluative words (e.g., "well," "good," "poorly," "bad")	Uses evaluative words (e.g., "good," "well," "excellent," "capably," "competent") more often
	Uses action statements (e.g., "You did ___, but you did not do ___," "I did not hear you ask ___," and "Another option would be ___")	
Most effective frequency	Often	Usually one-time event

lege Edition) tells us that *formative* means "susceptible of transformation by growth and development," while *summation*, the origin of the adverb *summative*, is "a concluding statement containing a summary of principal points." The primary differences between feedback and evaluation, elaborated on and applied to residency training, are given in Table 1. (Specific examples of feedback statements versus evaluation statements are presented in Table 2.) It becomes clear in examining these differences that feedback should be provided during a rotation or examination, whereas evaluation is intended for use after the rotation or examination has been completed.

Many barriers to providing useful feedback and to the overall evaluation process exist that may hinder a residency program's efforts to implement competency-based education and improvement of its curriculum over time. Most important among these barriers is the ever-increasing failure of supervising physicians, whether faculty or senior residents, to directly observe a learner's performance (Ende 1983). This is as true in clinic and hospital settings as it is in psychotherapy supervision. If there has been no observation of behavior, there will be no direct data on which to base an assessment. This lack of direct data makes it very difficult, if not impossible, to provide adequate and specific feedback. Moreover, it is this ongoing, specific, discrete feedback that fosters the development of competency over time. Therefore, basing feedback on scarce, inaccurate, or absent information will clearly create a flawed system for developing and assessing competency.

Table 2. Examples of feedback versus evaluation

Feedback	Evaluation
"You collected enough information to arrive at a diagnosis while establishing rapport with the patient."	"Your interviewing style is quite good."
"You did not know to monitor lithium levels in this patient when that would be an important part of managing his care."	"Your psychopharmacology knowledge is less advanced than that of other residents at your level of training."
"It is important that you recognized that your strong emotions in this case may have arisen from your difficult and competitive relationship with your father."	"You have an excellent grasp of the concepts, and real-world use of the theory, of transference and countertransference."
"You addressed all of the clinically important points regarding this patient except for alcohol use and family psychiatric history."	"Overall, that was a fine presentation."

With regard to "sit-down" rounds, or gatherings of teacher and learner(s) to discuss patients, many cognitive and dynamic-emotional impediments to accuracy exist for trainees' recall-based oral reports of patient interactions. A thorough discussion of that literature is beyond the scope of this volume. Recently, however, Tulsky and colleagues (2001) evaluated standardized patient interactions in which an observer faculty member, a standardized patient (SP), and the trainee interviewer were each asked to rate interpersonal skills and communication of the trainee during a standardized interview. Tulsky et al. found that there was a high degree of agreement between the faculty member and the SP in their ratings but a much lower degree of agreement between the trainee and the SP. This work suggests that trainees may have an inaccurate impression of their work with patients. The study also powerfully emphasizes the need for direct observation of trainees' work. Given the subjective nature of the work we do in psychiatry, direct observation and confirmation of learner reports are even more crucial to ensure accurate assessment of residents' work with patients.

The best way to collect data of trainees' work comes from repeated, in-person witnessing of complete patient interactions. However, this is probably not feasible for every situation or every faculty member. Alternatives to direct observation include

- Videotaped patient encounters.
- Audiotaped patient encounters.
- Process notes produced in session or from audiotapes.
- Observation of many, brief patient encounters or portions of patient interactions over time.

Time is another obstacle to adequate feedback and evaluation in psychiatric residency training. It takes considerable time and organization for a faculty member to provide ongoing, moment-to-moment feedback, formal midpoint feedback sessions, and final, summative written evaluation reviews for all trainees. To keep track of each individual's performance with specific examples, to distill one's thoughts from many weeks or even months of time on service, to provide thoughtful, kind, and productive information, and to complete the required paperwork can be an exhaustive and laborious process. This is particularly true if a faculty member hosts many trainees simultaneously throughout the year on his or her clinical service. It is worth remembering, as well, that the director of undergraduate education in the department is often asking simultaneously for similar input into the performance of many medical students on service.

It quickly becomes clear that the major investment of time and organizational skill involved with coordinating these many assessments is a significant barrier to their optimal implementation. One faculty member's tally of just midpoint and final feedback/evaluation sessions within the authors' training program helps to illustrate this point. Throughout the year, the attending hosted four medical students at a time on monthly rotations, two interns on monthly rotations, and four senior residents on quarterly rotations. The 144 midpoint and final feedback/evaluation sessions that this entailed would consume, conservatively (assuming 20 minutes per session to deliver and discuss feedback/evaluation as well as to receive same from trainee regarding faculty and rotation), 48 hours, or 6 full workdays, over the course of a year. Notably, this estimate of 48 hours does not include the time required to prepare one's written and verbal comments and to complete the paperwork. It is clear that a residency program that does not respect and acknowledge the deep commitment required from faculty to accomplish this crucial task of feedback and evaluation would undoubtedly struggle with implementing a competency-based curriculum.

The final barrier to feedback to be mentioned, and often the most powerful impediment, is the fear within both teacher and student that unintended and untoward consequences will result from the feedback or evaluation. Great potential exists for this process to elicit emotional reactions, particularly with the more final and subjective summative evaluations. There are many potential outcomes of feedback/evaluation, adverse and otherwise, but the greatest degree of trepidation, on the part of both teacher and learner, arises from the fear of a negative emotional reaction (Ende 1983; Klein and Babineau 1974) This fear leads to a number of potential concerns about the process:

- The learner may be hurt by the feedback/evaluation.
- The interaction might damage the learner-teacher relationship.
- The attending may be less popular as a result of giving negative feedback/evaluation. This may be a substantial issue in institutions where learners' ratings of faculty attendings are factored into promotion and compensation decisions, particularly if the faculty is asked to provide feedback to the learners before the learners have provided their evaluations.
- Learners will see feedback/evaluation statements as an indication of their personal value or worth.
- Learners may acknowledge feedback/evaluation only insofar as it confirms their self concept, leading to

devaluation of the feedback or of the teacher when discordance between feedback and self concept exists.

As important as acknowledging and respecting the time/organizational commitment required for effective feedback/evaluation, those in educational leadership positions would do well to recall the emotional difficulty inherent in the tasks we ask of our teachers and learners. According to Klein and Babineau (1974), the ego strengths required of both the educator and the trainee are "complex and difficult to integrate." A trainee is often expected to be simultaneously a naive student, responsible professional, sophisticated colleague, and friend, and, these authors might add, humble and grateful apprentice. Likewise, educators must be teacher, disciplinarian, character analyst, confidant, and decision-maker. These are no small accomplishments indeed. We have made progress over time, though, as Klein and Babineau (1974) remind us in noting "it is worth remembering that in medieval universities students were required to swear that if they did not succeed in their tests they would not 'take vengeance on the examiner with knife or other sharp instruments.'"

Understanding the Benefits of Multiple Assessments and Assessment Methods

In an ideal assessment system, as detailed within the ACGME Model Assessment System, multiple raters use a number of different assessment tools to make many ratings over a substantial period of time (Swing 2002). Clearly no single rating is able to provide the whole "truth" about a trainee's capacity to practice medicine with competence in the six general or five psychotherapy areas. A series of assessments from many different angles over a considerable length of time is required to fully paint the portrait of a resident's expertise. Patterns only emerge when a trainee is subjected to multiple assessments—an approach that diminishes the contribution of interpatient variability and poor interrater reliability (Epstein and Hundert 2002). This is axiomatic in the education literature and mandatory in planning an evaluation system within a residency program's curriculum.

Another important reason for using many different types of evaluation tools is the specificity of the different assessment instruments. Each of the six general competencies can be thought of as a collection of smaller tasks or skills, which have been called the "competency

components" and which in sum make up the greater general competency (Caraccio et al. 2002). To measure each of these components specifically and accurately presents academic psychiatry and medicine with a daunting task, perhaps even the "challenge of the decade" (Caraccio et al. 2002). It is illogical to think that it will require anything less than an elaborate battery of tests and measures to achieve this goal adequately. Therefore, each program must develop a repertoire of many assessment methods and assessors in order to capture data accurately on each of the competency components over time. A thorough discussion of many of the different assessment tools and their potential applicability can be found in Chapter 7 of this book. The ACGME Outcome Project Toolbox of Assessment Methods©, presented as an appendix to this chapter (see p. 23), describes many different assessment methods. Additionally, new tools are being developed continually—examples are the Strategic Management Simulation (Satish et al. 2001) and the Learning Plan (Taylor et al. 2002)—and many of these tools will become integral parts of the assessment batteries of residency programs over the coming decade and beyond.

This strategy of using multiple ratings can quickly become overly burdensome, since the "ultimate rating situation" could be one of infinite measurements applied daily by everyone involved with the learner. Clearly this process would exhaust all teaching faculty and residents and would be impossibly complex and laborious to administer (Leibrandt et al. 2001). Residency training directors and teaching faculty must always balance resident and faculty wear and tear against the needs of the educational program in order to maintain a positive and productive work and learning environment. This means that trade-offs will need to be made so that all the work of the day can proceed and yet sufficient data can be gathered to form an accurate and comprehensive picture of each resident's developing competence over time.

A substantial portion of the planning and effort expended in moving toward compliance with the ACGME competency requirements will be spent in determining which of the many available measures will be most effective when employed within a given residency program, who will be expected to complete these measures, and how often will they be completed. The work will be rewarded, hopefully, with a thorough and accurate assessment of each trainee's progress toward attaining competence as a physician, ready to practice medicine independently in the complex and ever-changing health care arena.

Matching Assessment Methods to Goals

The "gold standard" assessment instrument not only provides an accurate, reliable rating of a trainee's current performance but also predicts capacity for later quality in clinical practice and fosters future learning (Epstein and Hundert 2002). Additionally, the factors chosen for assessment will become surrogate representations of institutional values (Epstein and Hundert 2002), accentuating certain tasks or traits as standards and diminishing others by their omission. Therefore, considerable care should be employed in choosing assessment methods so that they will match the educational and philosophical goals of the residency program, fostering growth and development in trainees toward these chosen standards.

An example follows to illustrate the concept of matching assessments with goals. Consider a residency program that values interpersonal skill as the single most important component of psychiatric practice. If this residency program were to use multiple choice examinations as the predominate form of assessment, there would be a clear mismatch between assessment and goal, as performance on this type of exam has been shown to be inversely correlated with empathy (Tutton 1996). This example residency training program's mission and philosophy would be much better represented by the choice of Objective Structured Clinical Examinations (OSCEs) or Standardized Patient (SP) examinations to emphasize, teach, and evaluate residents' development of interpersonal skill competency.

The ACGME has constructed a resource, the Toolbox of Assessment Methods© (see appendix to this chapter), that lists, as well as describes in considerable detail, many different assessment methods. Residency program directors will likely find this toolbox to be helpful in deciding how to best match assessment methods to program goals.

"Teaching to the Test"

The phrase "teaching to the test" has almost become synonymous with inappropriate teaching practice in recent times. For the most part, this association stems from schools teaching to the high-stakes achievement testing employed in public schools with the often-inappropriate emphasis placed on student performance on these tests. In its most egregious form, "teaching to the test" in this sense means drilling students in rote memorization of actual test questions without instruction in the funda-

mental knowledge and background information necessary to understand concepts and skills represented by the questions. Generalization to new or ambiguous situations is almost impossible if teaching has focused solely or mostly on memorizing facts. The higher test scores among students taught in this fashion come at the expense of a broader knowledge and mastery of the full curriculum. The *concept* of "teaching to the test," however, is one that may be beneficial when exploited in the proper fashion. If used in this way, the test (or assessment instrument in the case of residency training) will emphasize certain knowledge or skill sets as being important and thereby emphasize that trainees demonstrate a minimum level of facility with that identified knowledge and skill set. The residency program's interest in *testing* the specified knowledge and skills will powerfully emphasize to residents and faculty the importance of teaching and developing competence in these specified areas.

"Curriculum teaching" is an example of appropriately teaching to the test in which teachers are required to direct their instruction toward a specific body of content knowledge or a specific set of cognitive skills represented by a given test (Popham 2001). This approach, which gives equal attention to all aspects of the body of knowledge or skill set, varies from the more problematic "item teaching," which emphasizes memorization of a specific set of answers to questions that will make up an examination. In curriculum teaching, a body of knowledge is mastered and competency is gained, whereas in item teaching, little appreciation of the origin of the answers is fostered and only a very crude capacity to manipulate the information is developed.

It is through this ability to manipulate previously learned information or skills in order to allow one to adapt to novel and ambiguous situations that competence has been defined (Epstein and Hundert 2002; Long 2000) One way to produce this type of learning is to design a curriculum that emphasizes breadth in learning and then to test for the desired principles within that body of knowledge or skill set. Learners will be taught to the test because faculty and trainees are very adaptable and will realize what is being measured. Therefore, returning to the beginning of this chapter, where it was noted, "You get what you measure," the tests (assessment measures) used in training will measure the educational objectives that have been prioritized, based on the educational philosophy of the given residency program. The faculty and trainees will progressively focus more, over time, on these very objectives, and the circular nature of testing, evaluating, modifying, and retesting will steer the curriculum ever nearer to the desired outcome. Physician competence is the desired outcome in the case of postgraduate psychiatric training. Residency training programs will "teach to the test" in the most appropriate fashion, and, in the words of the ACGME, "What you are measuring you will improve."

References

Caraccio C, Wolfsthal SD, Englander R, et al: Shifting paradigms: from Flexner to competencies. Acad Med 77(5): 361–367, 2002

Ende J: Feedback in clinical medical education. JAMA 250(6): 777–781, 1983

Epstein RM, Hundert EM: Defining and assessing professional competence. JAMA 287(2):226–235, 2002

Hensinger RN: Are we measuring the right things? J Pediatr Orthop 21(6):824–825, 2001

Klein RH, Babineau R: Evaluating the competence of trainees: it's nothing personal. Am J Psychiatry 131(7):788–791, 1974

Leibrandt TJ, Kukora JS, Dent TL: Integrating educational objectives and the evaluation process in a general surgery residency program. Acad Med 76(7):748–752, 2001

Long DM: Competency-based residency training: the next advance in graduate medical education. Acad Med 75(12): 1178–1183, 2000

Popham J: Teaching to the test. Educational Leadership 58(6), March 2001. Available at: http://www.ascd.org/readingroom/edlead/0103/popham.html. Accessed January 30, 2003.

Satish U, Streufert S, Marshall R, et al: Strategic management simulations is a novel way to measure resident competencies. Am J Surg 181(6):557–561, 2001

Swing S: Assessing the general competencies: ACGME Work in Progress. ACGME Bulletin, November 2002, pp 6–7

Taylor DK, Buterakos J, Campe J: Doing it well: demonstrating general competencies for resident education utilising the ACGME Toolbox of Assessment Methods as a guide for implementation of an evaluation plan. Med Educ 36: 1102–1103, 2002

Tulsky DS, Millis SR, Jain SS: Rating physician interpersonal skills: do patients and physicians see eye-to-eye. ACGME Outcome Project, 2001. Available at: http://www.acgme. org/outcome/implement/rsvpTemplate.asp?rsvpID=8. Accessed January 26, 2003.

Tutton PJ: Psychometric test results associated with high achievement in basic science components of medical education. Acad Med 71(2):181–186, 1996

Appendix

Toolbox of Assessment Methods©

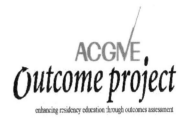

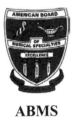

ABMS

TOOLBOX OF ASSESSMENT METHODS©

A Product of the Joint Initiative

ACGME Outcomes Project
Accreditation Council for Graduate Medical Education

American Board of Medical Specialties (ABMS)

Version 1.1
September 2000

TOOLBOX OF ASSESSMENT METHODS©

A Product of the Joint Initiative

ACGME Outcomes Project
Accreditation Council for Graduate Medical Education

American Board of Medical Specialties (ABMS)

Version 1.1
September 2000

Copyright Disclosure.

General Disclaimer.

The Toolbox includes descriptions of assessment methods that can be used for evaluating residents. It does not include all the tools that can or may be used by a residency program for evaluating residents, or by a program director in verifying that a resident has demonstrated sufficient professional ability to practice competently and independently. Neither ACGME nor ABMS shall be liable in any way for results obtained in applying these assessment methods. The user, and not ACGME or ABMS, shall be soley responsible for the results obtained in applying the assessment methods described herein. Further, the user agrees and acknowledges that, in using the Toolbox, he/she/it is solely responsible for complying with all applicable laws, regulations, and ordinances relating to privacy.

Table of Contents

ACGME/ABMS Joint Initiative
Toolbox of Assessment Methods
Version 1.1 September 2000
Page 1

Preface

Included in this packet are descriptions of assessment methods that can be used for evaluating residents. In addition to a brief description of each method, there is information pertaining to its use, psychometric qualities, and feasibility/practicality.

As a "work in progress," the descriptions reflect the most typical use and research findings related to the method. As this work proceeds, refinements and extensions that reflect the full potential and creative application of the methods can be expected.

The descriptions were developed to assist medical educators with the selection and development of evaluation techniques. They represent a first step in the construction of a more complete toolbox of assessment techniques.

The table on the last pages of this booklet rates assessment tools for robustness and practical use for assessing specific competencies expected of residents. The ratings are based upon a consensus of evaluation experts.

This work is supported in part by a grant from the Robert Wood Johnson Foundation to the Accreditation Council for Graduate Medical Education.

<table>
<tr><td>Susan Swing Ph.D.
ACGME Director of Research</td><td>Philip G. Bashook Ed.D.
ABMS Director of Evaluation and Education</td></tr>
</table>

ACGME/ABMS Joint Initiative
Toolbox of Assessment Methods
Version 1.1 September 2000
Page 2

Glossary

Generalizability – Measurements (scores) derived from an assessment tool are considered generalizable if they can be shown to apply to more than the sample of cases or test questions used in a specific assessment.

Reliability/Reproducibility – A reliable test score means when measurements (scores) are repeated the new test results are consistent with the first scores for the same assessment tool on the same or similar individuals. Reliability is measured as a correlation with 1.0 being perfect reliability and below 0.50 as unreliable. Evaluation measurement reliabilities above 0.65 and preferably near or above 0.85 are recommended.

Validity – Validating assessment measures is a process of accumulating evidence about how well the assessment measures represent or predict a resident's ability or behavior. Validity refers to the specific measurements made with assessment tools in a specific situation with a specific group of individuals. It is the scores not the type of assessment tool that are valid. For example, it is possible to determine if the written exam scores for a group of residents are valid in measuring the residents' knowledge, but it is incorrect to say that "all written exams" are valid to measure knowledge.

Formative Evaluation – In formative evaluation findings are accumulated from a variety of relevant assessments designed for use either in program or resident evaluation. In resident evaluation the formative evaluation is intended to provide constructive feedback to individual residents during their training. In program evaluation the formative evaluation is intended to improve program quality. In neither situation is formative evaluation intended to make a go/no-go decision.

Summative Evaluation – In summative evaluation findings and recommendations are designed to accumulate all relevant assessments for a go/no-go decision. In resident evaluation the summative evaluation is used to decide whether the resident qualifies to continue to the next training year, should be dropped from the program, or at the completion of the residency should be recommended for board certification. In program evaluation the summative evaluation is used to judge whether the program meets the accepted standards for the purpose of continuing, restructuring or discontinuing the program.

ACGME/ABMS Joint Initiative
Toolbox of Assessment Methods
Version 1.1 September 2000
Page 3

360-DEGREE EVALUATION INSTRUMENT

DESCRIPTION
360-degree evaluations consist of measurement tools completed by multiple people in a person's sphere of influence. Evaluators completing rating forms in a 360-degree evaluation usually are superiors, peers, subordinates, and patients and families. Most 360-degree evaluation processes use a survey or questionnaire to gather information about an individual's performance on several topics (e.g., teamwork, communication, management skills, decision-making). Most 360-degree evaluations use rating scales to assess how frequently a behavior is performed (e.g., a scale of 1 to 5, with 5 meaning "all the time" and 1 meaning "never"). The ratings are summarized for all evaluators by topic and overall to provide feedback.

USE
Evaluators provide more accurate and less lenient ratings when the evaluation is intended to give formative feedback rather than summative evaluations. A 360-degree evaluation can be used to assess interpersonal and communication skills, professional behaviors, and some aspects of patient care and systems-based practice.

PSYCHOMETRIC QUALITIES
No published reports of the use of 360-degree evaluation instruments in graduate medical education were found in the literature; however, there are reports of the use of various categories of people evaluating residents at the same time, although with different instruments.   Generally the evaluators were nurses, allied health professionals, other residents, faculty/supervisors, and patients.   Moderate correlations were found to exist among the scores produced by these evaluators using slightly different assessment tools. Reproducible results were most easily obtainable when five to ten nurses rated residents, while a greater number of faculty and patients were needed for the same degree of reliability. In business, military and education settings, reliability estimates have been reported as great as 0.90 for 360-degree evaluation instruments.

FEASIBILITY/PRACTICALITY
In most clinical settings conducting 360-degree-evaluations will pose a significant challenge. The two practical challenges are: constructing surveys that are appropriate for use by all evaluators in the circle of influence, and orchestrating data collection from a potentially large number of individuals that can be compiled and reported confidentially to the resident. Implementing an electronic system should make the 360-degree-evaluation feasible.

SUGGESTED REFERENCE
Center for Creative Leadership, Greensboro, North Carolina (http://www.ccl.org).

ACGME/ABMS Joint Initiative
Toolbox of Assessment Methods
Version 1.1 September 2000
Page 4

CHART STIMULATED RECALL ORAL EXAMINATION (CSR)

DESCRIPTION

In a chart stimulated recall (CSR) examination patient cases of the examinee (resident) are assessed in a standardized oral examination. A trained and experienced physician examiner questions the examinee about the care provided probing for reasons behind the work-up, diagnoses, interpretation of clinical findings, and treatment plans. The examiners rate the examinee using a well-established protocol and scoring procedure. In efficiently designed CSR oral exams each patient case (test item) takes 5 to 10 minutes. A typical CSR exam is two hours with one or two physicians as examiners per separate 30- or 60-minute session.

USE

These exams assess clinical decision-making and the application or use of medical knowledge with actual patients. Multiple-choice questions are better than CSR at assessing recall or understanding of medical knowledge. Five of the 24 ABMS Member Boards use CSR as part of their standardized oral examinations for initial certification.

PSYCHOMETRIC QUALITIES

Patient cases are selected to be a sample of patients the examinee should be able to manage successfully, for example, as a board certified specialist. One or more scores are derived for each case based upon pre-defined scoring rules. The examinee's performance is determined by combining scores from all cases for a pass/fail decision overall or by each session. If the CSR is used for certification, test scores are analyzed using sophisticated statistical methods (e.g., Item Response Theory (IRT) or generalizability theory) to obtain a better estimate of the examinee's ability. Exam score reliabilities have been reported between 0.65 and 0.88 (1.00 is considered perfect reliability). The physician examiners need to be trained in how to question the examinee and evaluate and score the examinee's responses.

FEASIBILITY/PRACTICALITY

"Mock orals," that use resident's cases but with much less standardization compared to board oral exams, often are used in residency training programs to help familiarize residents with the oral exams conducted for board certification. CSR oral exams can be implemented easily to determine if residents can apply knowledge appropriately in managing patients, but for the exams to be used for high stakes decisions about the resident's abilities such as board certification extensive resources and expertise are required to standardize the exam.

SUGGESTED REFERENCE

Munger, BS. Oral examinations. In Mancall EL, Bashook PG. (editors) *Recertification: new evaluation methods and strategies.* Evanston, Illinois: American Board of Medical Specialties, 1995: 39-42.

CHECKLIST EVALUATION

DESCRIPTION
Checklists consist of essential or desired specific behaviors, activities, or steps that make up a more complex competency or competency component. Typical response options on these forms are a check (☐) or "yes" to indicate that the behavior occurred or options to indicate the completeness (complete, partial, or absent) or correctness (total, partial, or incorrect) of the action. The forms provide information about behaviors but for the purpose of making a judgment about the adequacy of the overall performance, standards need to be set that indicate, for example, pass/fail or excellent, good, fair, or poor performance.

USE
Checklists are useful for evaluating any competency and competency component that can be broken down into specific behaviors or actions. Documented evidence for the usefulness of checklists exists for the evaluation of patient care skills (history and physical examination, procedural skills) and for interpersonal and communication skills. Checklists have also been used for self-assessment of practice-based learning skills (evidence-based medicine). Checklists are most useful to provide feedback on performance because checklists can be tailored to assess detailed actions in performing a task.

PSYCHOMETRIC QUALITIES
When observers are trained to use checklists, consistent scores can be obtained and reliability in the range of 0.7 to 0.8 is reported (1.0 is perfect reliability). Performance scores derived from checklists can discriminate between residents in different years of training. Scoring practitioners' behavior using checklists is more difficult when checklists assume a fixed sequence of actions because experienced physicians use various valid sequences and are usually parsimonious in their patient care behaviors.

FEASIBILITY/PRACTICALITY
To ensure validity of content and scoring rules, checklist development requires consensus by several experts with agreement on essential behaviors/actions, sequencing, and criteria for evaluating performance. Checklists require trained evaluators to observe performance and time to complete a checklist will vary depending on the observation period.

SUGGESTED REFERENCES
Noel G, Herbers JE, Caplow M, et al. How well do Internal Medicine faculty members evaluate the clinical skills of residents? *Ann Int Med*. 1992; 117: 757-65.

Winckel CP, Reznick RK, Cohen R, Taylor B. Reliability and construct validity of a structured technical skills assessment form. *Am J Surg.* 1994; 167: 423-27.

GLOBAL RATING OF LIVE OR RECORDED PERFORMANCE

DESCRIPTION

Global rating forms are distinguished from other rating forms in that (a) a rater judges general categories of ability (e.g., patient care skills, medical knowledge, interpersonal and communication skills) instead of specific skills, tasks or behaviors; and (b) the ratings are completed retrospectively based on general impressions collected over a period of time (e.g., end of a clinical rotation) derived from multiple sources of information (e.g., direct observations or interactions; input from other faculty, residents, or patients; review of work products or written materials). All rating forms contain scales that the evaluator uses to judge knowledge, skills, and behaviors listed on the form.   Typical rating scales consist of qualitative indicators and often include numeric values for each indicator, for example, (a) very good = 1, good =2, fair = 3, poor =4; or (b) superior =1, satisfactory =2, unsatisfactory =3. Written comments are important to allow evaluators to explain the ratings.

USE

Global rating forms are most often used for making end of rotation and summary assessments about performance observed over days or weeks. Scoring rating forms entails combining numeric ratings with comments to obtain a useful judgment about performance based upon more than one rater.

PSYCHOMETRIC QUALITIES

A number of problems with global ratings have been documented: scores can be highly subjective when raters are not well trained; sometimes all competencies are rated the same regardless of performance; and scores may be biased when raters inappropriately make severe or lenient judgments or avoid using the extreme ends of a rating scale. Research reports are mixed about: discriminating between competence levels of different individuals; rating more skilled/experienced physicians better than less experienced physicians; and reproducibility (reliability) of ratings by the same physician/faculty raters, across different physicians/faculty, and variability across physicians/faculty, residents, nurses, and patients ratings of the same resident.   Reproducibility appears easier to achieve for ratings of knowledge and more difficult to achieve for patient care and interpersonal and communication skills. A few studies have reported that faculty give more lenient ratings than residents, especially when the residents believe that the ratings will not be used for pass/fail decisions.

FEASIBILITY/PRACTICALITY

Basic global rating forms can be constructed and completed quickly and easily. However, ratings do require time to directly observe performance or interact with the physician being evaluated. Training of raters is important to improve reproducibility of the findings.

SUGGESTED REFERENCE

Gray J. Global rating scales in residency education. *Acad Med.* 1996; 71: S55-63.

ACGME/ABMS Joint Initiative
Toolbox of Assessment Methods
Version 1.1 September 2000
Page 7

OBJECTIVE STRUCTURED CLINICAL EXAMINATION (OSCE)

DESCRIPTION
In an objective structured clinical examination (OSCE) one or more assessment tools are administered at 12 to 20 separate standardized patient encounter stations, each station lasting 10-15 minutes. Between stations candidates may complete patient notes or a brief written examination about the previous patient encounter. All candidates move from station to station in sequence on the same schedule. Standardized patients are the primary assessment tool used in OSCEs, but OSCEs have included other assessment tools such as data interpretation exercises using clinical cases, and clinical scenarios with mannequins, to assess technical skills.

USE
OSCEs have been administered in most US medical schools, many residency programs, and by the licensure boards in Canada for more than five years. The OSCE format provides a standardized means to assess: physical examination and history taking skills; communication skills with patients and family members, breadth and depth of knowledge; ability to summarize and document findings; ability to make a differential diagnosis, or plan treatment; and clinical judgment based upon patient notes.

PSYCHOMETRIC QUALITIES
OSCEs can provide means to obtain direct measures in a standardized manner of a patient-doctor encounter. OSCEs are not useful to measure skills or abilities in continuity of care with repeated patient encounters or invasive procedures. Because OSCEs often use standardized patients the same advantages and limitations apply (see toolbox description of standardized patient examination). A separate performance score is derived for each task performed at a station and scores are combined across stations or tasks to determine a pass/fail score. Statistical weighting of scores on individual tasks is controversial and not recommended. An OSCE with 14 to 18 stations is recommended to obtain reliable measurements of performance.

FEASIBILITY/PRACTICALITY
OSCEs are very useful to measure specific clinical skills and abilities, but are difficult to create and administer. OSCEs are only cost-effective when many candidates are to be examined at one administration. Most OSCEs are administered in medical center outpatient facilities or specially designed patient examining rooms with closed circuit television. A separate room or cubical is needed for each station. For most residency programs developing and administering an OSCE will require the resources and expertise of a consortium of residency programs in an academic institution or metropolitan area.

SUGGESTED REFERENCE
Norman, Geoffrey. *Evaluation Methods: A resource handbook*. Hamilton, Ontario, Canada: Program for Educational Development, McMaster University, 1995: 71-77.

ACGME/ABMS Joint Initiative
Toolbox of Assessment Methods
Version 1.1 September 2000
Page 8

PROCEDURE, OPERATIVE, OR CASE LOGS

DESCRIPTION

Procedure, operative, or case logs document each patient encounter by medical conditions seen, surgical operation or procedures performed. The logs may or may not include counts of cases, operations, or procedures. Patient case logs currently in use involve recording of some number of consecutive cases in a designated time frame. Operative logs in current use vary; some entail comprehensive recording of operative data by CPT code while others require recording of operations or procedures for a small number of defined categories.

USE

Logs of types of cases seen or procedures performed are useful for determining the scope of patient care experience. Regular review of logs can be used to help the resident track what cases or procedures must be sought out in order to meet residency requirements or specific learning objectives. Patient logs documenting clinical experience for the entire residency can serve as a summative report of that experience; as noted below, the numbers reported do not necessarily indicate competence.

PSYCHOMETRIC QUALITIES

There are no known studies of case or procedure logs for the purpose of determining accuracy of residents' recording. Unless defined by CPT or other codes, cases or procedures counted for a given category may vary across residents and programs. Minimum numbers of procedures required for accreditation and certification have not been validated against the actual quality of performance of an operation or patient outcomes.

FEASIBILITY/PRACTICALITY

Electronic recording devices and systems facilitate the collection and summarization of patient cases or procedures performed. Although there is considerable cost associated with development, testing, and maintenance of electronic systems, these costs generally are not paid by individual programs and institutions, since systems are available commercially for a relatively small amount (e.g., $2500 annually) or provided free of charge by accrediting or certification bodies. Manual recording is required followed later by data entry unless automated data entry devices are located at or near the point of service. Data entry of manual records typically can be performed by a clerk, but is time consuming depending on the number of residents in the program and log reporting requirements.

SUGGESTED REFERENCE

Watts J, Feldman WB. Assessment of technical skills. In: Neufeld V and Norman G (ed). *Assessing clinical competence.* New York: Springer Publishing Company, 1985: 259-74.

PATIENT SURVEYS

DESCRIPTION

Surveys of patients to assess satisfaction with hospital, clinic, or office visits typically include questions about the physician's care. The questions often assess satisfaction with general aspects of the physician's care, (e.g., amount of time spent with the patient, overall quality of care, physician competency (skills and knowledge), courtesy, and interest or empathy). More specific aspects of care can be assessed including: the physician's explanations, listening skills and provision of information about examination findings, treatment steps, and drug side effects. A typical patient survey asks patients to rate their satisfaction with care using rating categories (e.g., poor, fair, good, very good, excellent) or agreement with statements describing the care (e.g., "the doctor kept me waiting," —Yes, always; Yes, sometimes; or No, never or hardly ever). Each rating is given a value and a satisfaction score calculated by averaging across responses to generate a single score overall or separate scores for different clinical care activities or settings.

USE

Patient feedback accumulated from single encounter questionnaires can assess satisfaction with patient care competencies (aspects of data gathering, treatment, and management; counseling, and education; preventive care); interpersonal and communication skills; professional behavior; and aspects of systems-based practice (patient advocacy; coordination of care). If survey items about specific physician behaviors are included, the results can be used for formative evaluation and performance improvement. Patient survey results also can be used for summative evaluation, but this use is contingent on whether the measurement process meets standards of reliability and validity.

PSYCHOMETRIC QUALITIES

Reliability estimates of 0.90 or greater have been achieved for most patient satisfaction survey forms used in hospitals and clinics. Reliability estimates are much lower for ratings of residents in training. The American Board of Internal Medicine reports 20-40 patient responses were needed to obtain a reliability of 0.70 to 0.82 on individual resident ratings using the ABIM Patient Satisfaction Questionnaire. Low per-resident reliability has been associated with surveys that use rating scales; survey questions with response options of "yes, definitely," "yes, somewhat," or "no," may provide more reproducible, and useful results.

FEASIBILITY/PRACTICALITY

A variety of patient satisfaction surveys are available from commercial developers and medical organizations. Creation of new surveys often begins with gathering input from patients using interviews, focus groups, or questionnaires. Physician attitudes and behaviors patients find to be satisfying or dissatisfying are then translated into survey items. Most patient satisfaction surveys are completed at the time of service, and require less than 10 minutes. Alternatively, they may be mailed after the patient goes home or conducted with patients over the phone. Difficulties encountered with patient surveys are: (1) language and

PATIENT SURVEYS

literacy problems; (2) obtaining enough per-resident surveys to provide reproducible results; (3) the resources required to collect, aggregate, and report survey responses; and
(4) assessment of the resident's contribution to a patient's care separate from that of the health care team. Because of these concerns, patient satisfaction surveys are often conducted by the institution or by one or more clinical sites and reports specific to the residency program may or may not be prepared. It may be possible to improve feasibility by utilizing effective survey design principles and using computers to collect and summarize survey data.

SUGGESTED REFERENCES

Kaplan SH, Ware JE. The patient's role in health care and quality assessment. In: Goldfield N and Nash D (eds). *Providing quality care (2nd ed): Future Challenge.* Ann Arbor, MI: Health Administration Press, 1995: 25-52.

Matthews DA, Feinstein AR. A new instrument for patients' ratings of physician performance in the hospital setting. *J Gen Intern Med.* 1989:4:14-22.

PORTFOLIOS

DESCRIPTION

A portfolio is a collection of products prepared by the resident that provides evidence of learning and achievement related to a learning plan. A portfolio typically contains written documents but can include video- or audio-recordings, photographs, and other forms of information. Reflecting upon what has been learned is an important part of constructing a portfolio. In addition to products of learning, the portfolio can include statements about what has been learned, its application, remaining learning needs, and how they can be met. In graduate medical education, a portfolio might include a log of clinical procedures performed; a summary of the research literature reviewed when selecting a treatment option; a quality improvement project plan and report of results; ethical dilemmas faced and how they were handled; a computer program that tracks patient care outcomes; or a recording or transcript of counseling provided to patients.

USE

Portfolios can be used for both formative and summative evaluation of residents. Portfolios are most useful for evaluating mastery of competencies that are difficult to evaluate in other ways such as practice-based improvement, use of scientific evidence in patient care, professional behaviors, and patient advocacy. Teaching experiences, morning report, patient rounds, individualized study or research projects are examples of learning experiences that lend themselves to using portfolios to assess residents. The Royal College of Physicians and Surgeons of Canada in the Maintenance of Competence Program (MOCOMPS) has developed a portfolio system for recertification using Internet-based diaries called PCDiary© that could be adapted to residency evaluations.

PSYCHOMETRIC QUALITIES

Reproducible assessments are feasible when there is agreement on criteria and standards for contents of a portfolio. When portfolio assessments have been used to evaluate an educational program (e.g., statewide elementary or high school program) the portfolio products or documentation have been found to be sufficient for program evaluation but are not always appropriate to use in assessing individual students for decisions about promotion to the next grade. However, standard criteria are not necessarily desirable and may be counter-productive when the portfolio purpose is to demonstrate individual learning gains relative to individual goals. The validity of portfolio assessment is determined by the extent to which the products or documentation included in a portfolio demonstrates mastery of expected learning.

FEASIBILITY/PRACTICALITY

Acceptance of portfolios in graduate medical education varies according to preferred learning style. Some residents and practicing physicians have found that by maintaining portfolios credit was allowed for some activities that otherwise would have gone undone or un-noticed. Yet, for others, the time and commitment necessary to create and maintain a portfolio is too great relative to the return.

SUGGESTED REFERENCE

Challis M. AMEE medical education guide no. 11 (revised): Portfolio-based learning and assessment in medical education. *Med Teach.* 1999; 21: 370-86.

ACGME/ABMS Joint Initiative
Toolbox of Assessment Methods
Version 1.1 September 2000
Page 12

RECORD REVIEW

DESCRIPTION

Trained staff in an institution's medical records department or clinical department perform a review of patients' paper or electronic records. The staff uses a protocol and coding form based upon predefined criteria to abstract information from the records, such as medications, tests ordered, procedures performed, and patient outcomes. The patient record findings are summarized and compared to accepted patient care standards. Standards of care are available for more than 1600 diseases on the Website of the Agency for HealthCare Research and Quality (http://www.ahrq.gov/).

USE

Record review can provide evidence about clinical decision-making, follow-through in patient management and preventive health services, and appropriate use of clinical facilities and resources (e.g., appropriate laboratory tests and consultations). Often residents will confer with other clinical team members before documenting patient decisions and therefore, the documented care may not be directly attributed to a single resident but to the clinical team.

PSYCHOMETRIC QUALITIES

A sample of approximately eight to 10 patient records is sufficient for a reliable assessment of care for a diagnosis or procedure. One study in office practice demonstrated that six to eight office records selected randomly are adequate to evaluate care. Missing or incomplete documentation of care is interpreted as not meeting the accepted standard.

FEASIBILITY/PRACTICALITY

Record reviews by trained staff take approximately 20 to 30 minutes per record on average for records of hospitalized patients. The major limitations are: (1) as a retrospective assessment of care the review may not be completed until sufficient patients have been treated which could delay reports about residents' performance for months after a typical one or two month clinical rotation; (2) criteria of care must be agreed-up and translated into coding forms for staff to review records; (3) staff must be trained in how to identify and code clinical data to assure reasonably reliable findings.

SUGGESTED REFERENCE

Tugwell P, Dok C. Medical record review. In: Neufeld V and Norman G (ed). *Assessing clinical competence.* New York: Springer Publishing Company, 1985: 142-82.

SIMULATIONS AND MODELS

DESCRIPTION

Simulations used for assessment of clinical performance closely resemble reality and attempt to imitate but not duplicate real clinical problems. Key attributes of simulations are that: they incorporate a wide array of options resembling reality, allow examinees to reason through a clinical problem with little or no cueing, permit examinees to make life-threatening errors without hurting a real patient, provide instant feedback so examinees can correct a mistaken action, and rate examinees' performance on clinical problems that are difficult or impossible to evaluate effectively in other circumstances. Simulation formats have been developed as paper-and-pencil branching problems (patient management problems or PMPs), computerized versions of PMPs called clinical case simulations (CCX®), role-playing situations (e.g., standardized patients [SPs], clinical team simulations), anatomical models or mannequins, and combinations of all three formats. Mannequins are imitations of body organs or anatomical body regions frequently using pathological findings to simulate patient disease. The models are constructed of vinyl or plastic sculpted to resemble human tissue with imbedded electronic circuitry to allow the mannequin to respond realistically to actions by the examinee. Virtual reality simulations or environments (VR) use computers sometimes combined with anatomical models to mimic as much as feasible realistic organ and surface images and the touch sensations (computer generated haptic responses) a physician would expect in a real patient. The VR environments allow assessment of procedural skills and other complex clinical tasks that are difficult to assess consistently by other assessment methods.

USE

Simulations using VR environments have been developed to train and assess surgeons performing arthroscopy of the knee and other large joints, anesthesiologists managing life-threatening critical incidents during surgery, surgeons performing wound debridement and minor surgery, and medical students and residents responding to cardio-pulmonary incidents on a full-size human mannequin. Written and computerized simulations have been used to assess clinical reasoning, diagnostic plans and treatment for a variety of clinical disciplines as part of licensure and certification examinations. Standardized patients as simulations are described elsewhere.

PSYCHOMETRIC QUALITIES

Studies of high-quality simulations have demonstrated their content validity when the simulation is designed to resemble a real patient. One or more scores are derived for each simulation based upon pre-defined scoring rules set by the experts in the discipline. The examinee's performance is determined by combining scores from all simulations to derive an overall performance score. When included in Objective Structured Clinical Examinations (OSCEs) the case reliabilities are similar to those reported for OSCEs (See OSCEs).

FEASIBILITY/PRACTICALITY

Experts in a specialty carefully craft simulations as clinical scenarios from real patient cases to focus the assessments on specific skills, abilities and "key features" of the case. Technical experts in assessment and simulations then convert the scenarios into simulations as standardized patients, mannequins,

ACGME/ABMS Joint Initiative
Toolbox of Assessment Methods
Version 1.1 September 2000
Page 14

SIMULATIONS AND MODELS

computer-based simulations, and other simulations adding when feasible computer-automated scoring rules to record the examinees' actions. Simulations are expensive to create and often require producing many variations of the pathological conditions or clinical problems to make them economical.   Grants and contracts from commercial vendors, foundations, governmental agencies and medical schools continue to be the principle source of funding to develop simulations.

SUGGESTED REFERENCE
Tekian A, McGuire CH, et al. (eds.) *Innovative simulations for assessing professional competence.* Chicago, Illinois: University of Illinois at Chicago, Dept. Med. Educ. 1999

STANDARDIZED ORAL EXAMINATION

DESCRIPTION

The standardized oral examination is a type of performance assessment using realistic patient cases with a trained physician examiner questioning the examinee. The examiner begins by presenting to the examinee a clinical problem in the form of a patient case scenario and asks the examinee to manage the case. Questions probe the reasoning for requesting clinical findings, interpretation of findings, and treatment plans. In efficiently designed exams each case scenario takes three to five minutes. Exams last approximately 90 minutes to two and one-half hours with two to four separate 30- or 60-minute sessions. One or two physicians serve as examiners per session. An examinee can be tested on 18 to 60 different clinical cases.

USE

These exams assess clinical decision-making and the application or use of medical knowledge with realistic patients. Multiple-choice questions are better at assessing recall or understanding of medical knowledge. Fifteen of the 24 ABMS Member Boards use standardized oral examinations as the final examination for initial certification.

PSYCHOMETRIC QUALITIES

A committee of experts in the specialty carefully crafts the clinical scenarios from real patient cases to focus the assessment on the "key features" of the case. Cases are selected to be a sample of patients the examinee should be able to manage successfully, for example, as a board certified specialist. One or more scores are derived for each case based upon pre-defined scoring rules. The examinee's performance is determined by combining scores from all cases for a pass/fail decision overall or by each session. Test scores are analyzed using sophisticated statistical methods (e.g., Item Response Theory [IRT] or generalizability theory) to obtain a better estimate of the examinee's ability. Exam score reliabilities have been reported between 0.65 and 0.88 (1.00 is considered perfect reliability). The physician examiners need to be trained in how to provide patient data for each scenario, question the examinee, and evaluate and score the examinee's responses.

FEASIBILITY/PRACTICALITY

A committee of physician specialists develops the examination cases and trains the examiners, often with assistance from psychometric experts. "Mock orals," that use cases but with much less standardization compared to board oral exams, are often used in residency training programs to help familiarize residents with the oral exams conducted for board certification. Extensive resources and expertise are required, however, to develop and administer a standardized oral examination.

SUGGESTED REFERENCE

Mancall EL, Bashook PG. (eds.) *Assessing clinical reasoning: the oral examination and alternative methods*. Evanston, Illinois: American Board of Medical Specialties, 1995.

STANDARDIZED PATIENT EXAMINATION (SP)

DESCRIPTION

Standardized patients (SPs) are well persons trained to simulate a medical condition in a standardized way or actual patients who are trained to present their condition in a standardized way. A standardized patient exam consists of multiple SPs each presenting a different condition in a 10-12 minute patient encounter. The resident being evaluated examines the SP as if (s)he were a real patient, (i.e., the resident might perform a history and physical exam, order tests, provide a diagnosis, develop a treatment plan, or counsel the patient). Using a checklist or a rating form, a physician observer or the SPs evaluate the resident's performance on appropriateness, correctness, and completeness of specific patient care tasks and expected behaviors (see description of Checklist Evaluation…). Performance criteria are set in advance. Alternatively or in addition to evaluation using a multiple SP exam, individual SPs can be used to assess specific patient care skills. SPs are also included as stations in Objective Structured Clinical Examinations (see description of OSCE).

USE

SPs have been used to assess history-taking skills, physical examination skills, communication skills, differential diagnosis, laboratory utilization, and treatment. Reproducible scores are more readily obtained for history-taking, physical examination, and communication skills. Standardized patient exams are most frequently used as summative performance exams for clinical skills. A single SP can assess targeted skills and knowledge.

PSYCHOMETRIC QUALITIES

Standardized patient examinations can generate reliable scores for individual stations and total performance useful for pass-fail decisions. Training of raters whether physicians, patients or other types of observers is critical to obtain reliable scores. At least one-half day of testing time (four hours) is needed to obtain reliable scores for assessment of hands-on clinical skills. Research on the validity of some SP exams has found better performance by senior residents than junior residents (construct validity) and modest correlations between SP exam scores and clinical ratings or written exams (concurrent validity).

FEASIBILITY/PRACTICALITY

Development of an examination using standardized patients involves identification of the specific competencies to be tested, training of standardized patients, development of checklists or rating forms and criteria setting. Development time can be considerable, but can be made more time efficient by sharing of SPs in a collaboration of multiple residency programs or in a single academic medical center. A new SP can learn to stimulate a new clinical problem in

STANDARDIZED PATIENT EXAMINATION (SP)

8 to 10 hours; and an experienced SP can learn a new problem in 6 to 8 hours. About twice the training time is needed for SPs to learn to use checklists to evaluate resident performance. Facilities needed for the examination include an examining room for each SP station and space for residents to record medical notes between stations.

SUGGESTED REFERENCE
Van der Vleuten CPM, and Swanson D. Assessment of clinical skills with standardized patients: State of the art. *Teach Learn Med*. 1990; 2: 58-76.

ACGME/ABMS Joint Initiative
Toolbox of Assessment Methods
Version 1.1 September 2000
Page 18

WRITTEN EXAMINATION (MCQ)

DESCRIPTION

A written or computer-based MCQ examination is composed of multiple-choice questions (MCQ) selected to sample medical knowledge and understanding of a defined body of knowledge, not just factual or easily recalled information. Each question or test item contains an introductory statement followed by four or five options in outline format. The examinee selects one of the options as the presumed correct answer by marking the option on a coded answer sheet. Only one option is keyed as the correct response. The introductory statement often presents a patient case, clinical findings, or displays data graphically. A separate booklet can be used to display pictures, and other relevant clinical information. The in-training examinations prepared by specialty societies and boards use MCQ type test items. A typical half-day examination has 175 to 250 test questions.

In computer-based examinations the test items are displayed on a computer monitor one at a time with pictures and graphical images also displayed directly on the monitor. In a computer-adaptive test fewer test questions are needed because test items are selected based upon statistical rules programmed into the computer to quickly measure the examinee's ability.

USE

Medical knowledge and understanding can be measured by MCQ examinations. Comparing the test scores on in-training examinations with national statistics can serve to identify strengths and limitations of individual residents to help them improve. Comparing test results aggregated for residents in each year of a program can be helpful to identify residency training experiences that might be improved.

PSYCHOMETRIC QUALITIES

For test questions to be useful in evaluating a resident's knowledge each test item and the overall exam should be designed to rigorous psychometric standards. Psychometric qualities must be high for pass/fail decisions, but tests used to help residents identify strengths and weaknesses such as in-training examinations need not comply with the same rigorous standards. A committee of experts designing the test defines the knowledge to be assessed and creates a test blueprint that specifies the number of test questions to be selected for each topic. When test questions are used to make pass/fail decisions the test should be pilot tested and statistically analyzed. A higher reliability/reproducibility can be achieved with more test questions per topic. If pass/fail decisions will be made based on test scores a sufficient number of test questions should be included to obtain a test reliability greater than r = 0.85 (1.00 is perfect reliability). Standards for passing scores should be set by a committee of experts prior to administering the examination (criterion referenced exams). If performance of residents is to be compared from year to year at least 25 to 30 percent of the same test questions should be repeated each year.

Toolbox of Assessment Methods© 2000 Accreditation Council for Graduate Medical Education (ACGME), and American Board of Medical Specialties (ABMS). Version 1.1.

WRITTEN EXAMINATION (MCQ)

FEASIBILITY/PRACTICALITY

A committee of physician specialists develops the examination with assistance from psychometric experts. For in-training examinations each residency program administers an exam purchased from the specialty society or other vendor. Tests are scored by the vendor and scores returned to the residency director for each resident, for each topic, and by year of residency training. Comparable national scores also are provided. All the 24 ABMS Member Boards use MCQ examinations for initial certification.

SUGGESTED REFERENCES

Haladyna TM. *Developing and validating multiple-choice test items*. Hillsdale, New Jersey: L. Erlbaum Associates. 1994.

Case SM, Swanson DB. *Constructing written test questions for the basic and clinical sciences*. Philadelphia, PA: National Board of Medical Examiners, 1996 (www.nbme.org).

List of Suggested References

Case SM, Swanson DB. *Constructing written test questions for the basic and clinical sciences.* Philadelphia, PA: National Board of Medical Examiners, 1996 (www.nbme.org).

Center for Creative Leadership, Greensboro, North Carolina (http://www.ccl.org).

Challis M. AMEE medical education guide no. 11 (revised): Portfolio-based learning and assessment in medical education. *Med Teach.* 1999; 21: 370-86.

Gray, J. Global rating scales in residency education. *Acad Med.* 1996; 71: S55-63.

Haladyna TM. *Developing and validating multiple-choice test items.* Hillsdale, New Jersey: L. Erlbaum Associates. 1994.

Kaplan SH, Ware JE. The patient's role in health care and quality assessment. In: Goldfield N and Nash D (eds). *Providing quality care (2nd ed): Future Challenge.* Ann Arbor, MI: Health Administration Press, 1995: 25-52.

Matthews DA, Feinstein AR. A new instrument for patients' ratings of physician performance in the hospital setting. *J Gen Intern Med.* 1989:4:14-22.

Mancall EL, Bashook PG. (eds.) *Assessing clinical reasoning: the oral examination and alternative methods.* Evanston, Illinois: American Board of Medical Specialties, 1995.

Munger, BS. Oral examinations. In Mancall EL, Bashook PG. (editors) *Recertification: new evaluation methods and strategies.* Evanston, Illinois: American Board of Medical Specialties, 1995: 39-42.

Noel G, Herbers JE, Caplow M, et al. How well do Internal Medicine faculty members evaluate the clinical skills of residents? *Ann Int Med.* 1992; 117: 757-65.

Norman, Geoffrey. *Evaluation Methods: A resource handbook.* Hamilton, Ontario, Canada: Program for Educational Development, McMaster University, 1995: 71-77.

Tekian A, McGuire CH, et al. (eds.) *Innovative simulations for assessing professional competence.* Chicago, Illinois: University of Illinois at Chicago, Dept. Med. Educ. 1999.

Tugwell P, Dok C. Medical record review. In: Neufeld V and Norman G (ed). *Assessing clinical competence.* New York: Springer Publishing Company, 1985: 142-82.

Van der Vleuten, CPM and Swanson, D. Assessment of clinical skills with standardized patients: State of the art. *Teach Learn Med.* 1990; 2: 58-76.

Watts J, Feldman WB. Assessment of technical skills. In: Neufeld V and Norman G (ed). *Assessing clinical competence.* New York: Springer Publishing Company, 1985, 259-74.

Winckel CP, Reznick RK, Cohen R, Taylor B. Reliability and construct validity of a structured technical skills assessment form. *Am J Surg.* 1994; 167: 423-27.

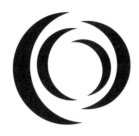

Part III

Implementing the General and Psychotherapy Competencies

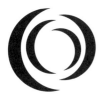

5

Defining Knowledge, Skills, and Attitudes to Be Taught for Each General Competency

Defining what is meant by competency, let alone what amounts to competency within each of the six general areas identified by the ACGME, has proven to be a substantial challenge in the implementation of the new standards. Though the ACGME itself offers no definition of competency within the Outcome Project or Program Requirements, several definitions have been offered elsewhere. Examples include

> Having requisite or adequate ability or qualities. (*Webster's New Collegiate Dictionary*)

> [T]he habitual and judicious use of communication, knowledge, technical skills, clinical reasoning, emotions, values, and reflection in daily practice for the benefit of the individual and community being served. (Epstein and Hundert 2002)

> [A] complex set of behaviors built on the components of knowledge, skills, attitudes, and 'competence' as personal ability. (Caraccio et al. 2002)

What follows within this chapter is an attempt to bring these definitions to bear on each of the ACGME's six General Competencies: Patient Care, Medical Knowledge, Practice-Based Learning and Improvement, Interpersonal and Communication Skills, Professionalism, and Systems-Based Practice. Example components of each competency will be included, as well as a discussion of the nature of each competency. The majority of the

information comes directly from the ACGME itself and can be found in the Outcome Project portion of the ACGME website (www.acgme.org/Outcome).

Patient Care

The Outcome Project includes language stating that "residents must be able to provide patient care that is compassionate, appropriate, and effective for the treatment of health problems and the promotion of health." This particular competency is dependent on a number of the other five competencies to a unique degree. It is hard to imagine a skilled clinician delivering compassionate care without some degree of competence in interpersonal and communication skills. Likewise, appropriate, effective decisions must be based on adequate medical knowledge. Patient care as a competency, however, combines many of the other competencies into a broader category wherein effective application toward management of the patient is the key outcome. For example, a resident might be tremendously interpersonally gifted and perform quite capably on tests of medical knowledge but still fail to coordinate these skills in such a way that patients are cared for with compassion, appropriateness, and effectiveness.

The ACGME's list of the expectations subsumed under the heading of Patient Care includes that a competent resident should be able to do the following:

- Communicate effectively and demonstrate caring and respectful behaviors when interacting with patients and their families.
- Gather essential and accurate information about their patients.
- Make informed decisions about diagnostic and therapeutic interventions based on patient information and preferences, up-to-date scientific evidence, and clinical judgment.
- Develop and carry out patient management plans.
- Counsel and educate patients and families.
- Use information technology to support patient care decisions and patient education.
- Perform competently all medical and invasive procedures considered essential for the area of practice.
- Provide healthcare services aimed at preventing health problems or maintaining health.
- Work with healthcare professionals, including those from other disciplines, to provide patient-focused care.

In concert with the American Association of Directors of Psychiatric Residency Training (AADPRT), prominent psychiatric educators developed a comprehensive and extensive list of psychiatry-specific competencies within the six General Competencies. Gene Beresin, M.D., Glenn Davis, M.D., John Herman, M.D., and Andrews Russell, M.D., coordinated these development efforts. Their outline of the psychiatry-specific components for the Patient Care General Competency follows.

1. The resident shall demonstrate the ability to perform and document a comprehensive psychiatric history examination of culturally diverse adult, geriatric, and child/adolescent patients to include

   - Complete present and past psychiatric history.
   - Sociocultural and educational history.
   - Family history, including ethnocultural and generational aspects.
   - Substance abuse history.
   - Medical history and review of systems.
   - Physical and neurological examination.
   - Comprehensive and mental status examination, including the assessment of cognitive functioning.
   - Developmental history.

2. Based on a comprehensive psychiatric assessment (see no. 1 above), the resident shall demonstrate the ability to develop and document

   - Complete DSM multiaxial differential diagnosis.

   - Integrative case formulation that includes neurobiological, phenomenological, psychological, and sociocultural issues involved in diagnosis and management.
   - Evaluation plan, including appropriate laboratory, medical, and psychological examinations.
   - Comprehensive treatment plan addressing biological and sociocultural domains.

3. The resident shall demonstrate the ability to comprehensively assess, discuss, and document the patients' potential for self-harm or harm to others and to intervene. This ability shall include

   - Assessment of risk based on known risk factors.
   - Knowledge of involuntary treatment standards and procedures.
   - Effective intervention to minimize risk.
   - Implementation of prevention methods for self-harm and harm to others.

4. The resident shall demonstrate the ability to conduct therapeutic interviews (e.g., enhance the ability to collect and use clinically relevant material through the conduct of supportive interventions) and to carry out exploratory interventions and clarifications.

5. The resident shall demonstrate the ability to conduct a range of individual, group, and family therapies, using standard, accepted models that are evidence-based, and integrate these psychotherapies in multimodel treatment, including biological and sociocultural interventions.

Medical Knowledge

Medical Knowledge is perhaps the most readily understandable and quantifiable of the competencies, and, along with timed requirements, the one that has been the focus of medical education since the era of the Flexner Report. Clearly, the competent practitioner must have a broad, current, and accurate foundation of knowledge in his or her area of practice in order to diagnose and treat medical illness adequately. The ACGME stipulates, "Residents must demonstrate knowledge about established and evolving biomedical, clinical, and cognate . . . sciences and the application of this knowledge to patient care." Succinctly outlined within the Outcome Project, this includes

- Demonstrating an investigatory and analytic thinking approach to clinical decisions.

- Knowing and applying the basic and clinically supportive sciences which are appropriate to their discipline.

The outline of the psychiatry-specific components of the Medical Knowledge General Competency, as developed by Drs. Beresin, Davis, Herman, and Russell, follows.

1. The resident shall demonstrate knowledge of the major psychiatric disorders, including age, gender, and sociocultural considerations, based on the scientific literature and standards of practice. This knowledge shall include

    - Epidemiology of the disorder.
    - Etiology of the disorder, including (when known) medical, genetic, and sociocultural factors.
    - Phenomenology of the disorder.
    - Experience, meaning, and explanation of the illness for the patient and family, including the influence of cultural factors and culture-bound syndromes.
    - DSM diagnostic criteria.
    - Effective treatment strategies.
    - Course and prognosis.

2. The resident shall demonstrate knowledge of psychotropic medications, including the antidepressants, antipsychotics, anxiolytics, mood stabilizers, hypnotics, and stimulants. This knowledge shall include

    - Pharmacological action.
    - Clinical indications.
    - Side effects.
    - Drug interactions (including over-the-counter, herbal, and alternative medications).
    - Toxicity.
    - Appropriate prescribing practices.
    - Age, gender, and ethnocultural variations.

3. The resident shall demonstrate knowledge of substances of abuse. This knowledge shall include

    - Pharmacological action.
    - Signs and symptoms of toxicity.
    - Signs and symptoms of tolerance and withdrawal.
    - Management of toxicity, tolerance, and withdrawal.
    - Epidemiology, including sociocultural factors.

4. The resident shall demonstrate knowledge of human growth and development, including normal biological, cognitive, and psychosexual development, including sociocultural, economic, ethnic, gender, religious/spiritual, sexual orientation, and family factors.

5. The resident shall demonstrate knowledge of emergency psychiatry. This knowledge shall include

    - Suicide.
    - Crisis intervention.
    - Differential diagnosis in emergency situations.
    - Treatment methods in emergency situations.
    - Homicide, rape, and violent behavior.

6. The resident shall demonstrate knowledge of behavioral science and sociocultural psychiatry. This knowledge shall include

    - Learning theory.
    - Theories of normal family organization, dynamics, and communication.
    - Theories of groups dynamic and process.
    - Theology, anthropology, and sociology as they pertain to clinical psychiatry.
    - Transcultural psychiatry.
    - Community mental health.
    - Epidemiology.
    - Research methods and statistics.

7. The resident shall demonstrate knowledge of psychosocial therapies. This knowledge shall include

    - All forms of psychotherapies (group, individual, family, behavioral theory and practice).
    - Treatments of psychosexual dysfunctions.
    - Hypnosis.
    - Doctor-patient relationship.

8. The resident shall demonstrate knowledge of somatic treatment methods. This knowledge shall include

    - Pharmacotherapy (as indicated in no. 2 earlier in this list).
    - ECT.
    - Biofeedback.

9. The resident shall demonstrate knowledge of patient evaluation and treatment selection. This knowledge shall include

    - Psychological testing.
    - Laboratory methods used in psychiatry.
    - Mental status examination.
    - Diagnostic interviewing.
    - Treatment comparison and selection.

10. The resident shall demonstrate knowledge of consultation-liaison psychiatry. This knowledge shall include

    - Specific syndromes (e.g., stress reactions, postpartum disorders, pain syndromes, postsurgical and ICU reactions).
    - Psychiatric aspects of nonpsychiatric illness.
    - Psychiatric complications of nonpsychiatric treatment.
    - Psychosomatic and somatopsychic disorders.
    - Models of consultation psychiatry.

11. The resident shall demonstrate knowledge in child and adolescent psychiatry. This knowledge shall include

    - Assessment and treatment of children and adolescents.
    - Disorders usually first diagnosed in infancy, childhood or adolescence.
    - Mental retardation and other developmental disabilities.

12. The resident shall demonstrate knowledge in forensic psychiatry.
13. The resident shall demonstrate knowledge in administrative psychiatry and in systems of health-care delivery.
14. The resident shall demonstrate knowledge of ethics.

Practice-Based Learning and Improvement

The ability to learn from day-to-day experience and avoid repetitive errors is delineated within this competency. Recent activity within the RRC Outcome Project Think Tank has offered additional guidance about the expectations of the ACGME with regard to practice-based learning (Swing 2002). Although not prescription, but guidance, this new information will prove valuable in fashioning a residency program that adequately addresses education in this competency area. The RRC Outcome Project Think Tank group emphasized that "residents must internalize the value of ongoing, self-directed learning and improvement of practice and that this would be demonstrated when residents: (a) reflect on and analyze practice experience; (b) locate and apply scientific evidence; (c) take steps to improve practice; and (d) demonstrate improvements."

Within the original wording of the ACGME Outcome Project, "residents must be able to investigate and evaluate their patient care practices, appraise and assimilate scientific evidence, and improve their patient care practices." This includes residents' ability to

- Analyze practice experience and perform practice-based improvement activities using systematic methodology.
- Locate, appraise, and assimilate evidence from scientific studies related to their patients' health problems.
- Obtain and use information about their own population of patients and the larger population from which their patients are drawn.
- Apply knowledge of study designs and statistical methods to the appraisal of clinical studies and other information on diagnostic and therapeutic effectiveness.
- Use information technology to manage information, access on-line medical information, and support their own education.
- Facilitate the learning of students and other health-care professionals.

The outline of the psychiatric-specific components of the Practice-Based Learning and Improvement General Competency, as developed by Drs. Beresin, Davis, Herman, and Russell, follows.

1. Psychiatrists must recognize and accept limitations in one's knowledge base and clinical skills, and understand the need for lifelong learning.
2. The resident will have appropriate skills and demonstrate obtaining up-to-date information from the scientific and practice literature and other sources to assist in the quality care of patients. These shall include but not be limited to

    - Use of medical libraries.
    - Use of information technology, including Internet-based searches and literature databases (e.g., Medline).
    - Use of drug information databases.

3. The resident shall evaluate caseload and practice experience in a systematic manner. This evaluation may include

    - Maintaining patient logs.
    - Reviewing patient records and outcomes.
    - Obtaining evaluations from patients and family members (e.g., outcomes and patient/family satisfaction).
    - Obtaining appropriate supervision and consultation.

- Maintaining a system for examining errors in practice and initiating improvements to eliminate or reduce errors.

4. The resident shall demonstrate an ability to critically evaluate the psychiatric literature. This ability may include

- Using knowledge of common methodologies employed in psychiatric research to evaluate studies, particularly drug treatment trials.
- Conducting and presenting reviews of current research in such formats as journal clubs, grand rounds, and/or original publications.
- Researching and summarizing a particular problem that derives from the resident's caseload.

5. The resident shall be able to

- Review and critically assess the scientific literature to determine how quality of care can be improved in relation to one's practice (i.e., reliable and valid assessment techniques, treatment approaches with established effectiveness, practice parameter adherence). Within this aim, the resident should be able to assess the generalizability or applicability of research findings to one's patients, in relation to their sociocultural and clinical characteristics.
- Develop and pursue effective remediation strategies based on critical review of the scientific literature.

Interpersonal and Communication Skills

Elemental in any specialty of medicine, the ability to communicate and develop interpersonal rapport with patients is of critical importance to the practice of psychiatry. These qualities have also been delineated under the rubric of "humanism" (Misch 2002), but, by any name, the attitudes, skills, and behaviors that create strong interpersonal ability are integral to the effective practice of medicine.

According to the ACGME, "Residents must be able to demonstrate interpersonal and communication skills that result in effective information exchange and teaming with patients, their patients' families, and professional associates." This includes the following important skills:

- Create and sustain a therapeutic and ethically sound relationship with patients.

- Use effective listening skills and elicit and provide information using effective nonverbal, explanatory, questioning, and writing skills.
- Work effectively with others as a member or leader of a healthcare team or other professional group.

The outline of the psychiaty-specific components of the Interpersonal and Communication Skills General Competency, as developed by Drs. Beresin, Davis, Herman, and Russell, follows.

1. Interpersonal skills refer to the ability of the psychiatrist to develop and maintain therapeutic relationships with culturally diverse patients and work collaboratively with professionals and the public.
2. Interpersonal skills require an underlying attitude of respect for others (including those with differing points of view or from culturally diverse backgrounds), the desire to gain understanding of another's position and reasoning, a belief in the intrinsic worth of all human beings, the wish to build collaboration, the desire to share information in a consultative rather than in an dogmatic fashion, and the willingness to continuously self-observe and confront one's own biases and transferences.
3. Interpersonal skills are defined as the specific techniques and methods that facilitate effective and emphatic communication between the psychiatrist, patients, families, significant others, colleagues, staff, and healthcare system.
4. The competent resident can demonstrate the ability to

- Listen to and understand patients and families.
- Communicate effectively with patients and families, using verbal, nonverbal, and writing skills as appropriate.
- Foster a therapeutic alliance with patients, as indicated by instilling feelings of trust, openness, rapport, and comfort in the relationship with the physician.
- Use negotiation to develop an agreed upon healthcare management plan with patients and families when appropriate.
- Transmit information to patients and families in a clear, meaningful fashion.
- Understand the impact of the physician's feelings and behavior on psychiatric treatment.
- Communicate effectively with allied healthcare professionals and with other professionals involved in the life of patients.

- Educate patients, families, and professionals about medical, psychological, and behavioral issues.
- Work effectively within multidisciplinary team structures as member, consultant, or leader.
- Form relationships with patients, families, and professionals in a culturally sensitive and responsive fashion.
- Exhibit professional, ethically sound behavior and attitudes in all patient and professional interactions.

5. The resident shall demonstrate the ability to elicit information. This will include skills in eliciting important diagnostic data and data affecting treatment from individuals from culturally diverse backgrounds as well as skills in tolerating and managing high levels of affect in the patients.

6. The resident shall demonstrate the ability to obtain, interpret, and evaluate consultations from other medical specialties, other helping professionals, and community-based resources. This ability shall include

- Formulating and clearly communicating the consultation question.
- Discussing the consultation findings with the consultation.
- Evaluating the consultation findings.

7. The resident shall serve as an effective consultant to other medical specialists, mental health and other helping professionals, and community-based resources. The resident should demonstrate the ability to

- Communicate effectively with the requesting party to refine the consultation question.
- Maintain the role of consultant.
- Communicate clear and specific recommendations.
- Respect the knowledge and expertise of the requesting party.

8. The resident shall demonstrate the ability to communicate effectively with patients and their families and significant others by

- Providing explanations of psychiatric disorders and treatment (both verbally and in written form) that are jargon free and geared to their educational/intellectual level.
- Providing preventive education that is understandable and practical.

- Respecting the patient's and family's cultural, ethnic, and economic background and identity and its impact on the illness of experience, meaning, and explanation.
- Demonstrating the ability to develop and enhance rapport and a working alliance with patients, families, and significant others.

9. The resident shall demonstrate the ability to manage his or her own affects and countertransference. This will include the cross-cultural context, which might involve bias and stereotyping.

10. The resident shall maintain psychiatric medical records that are

- Legible.
- Timely.
- Able to capture essential information useful to nonpsychiatric health professionals while simultaneously respecting patient privacy.

11. The resident shall demonstrate the ability to effectively lead a multidisciplinary treatment team. This skill includes the ability to

- Listen effectively.
- Elicit needed information from team members.
- Integrate information from different disciplines.
- Manage conflict.
- Clearly communicate an integrated treatment plan respecting the sociocultural diversity of the team members.

12. The resident shall demonstrate the ability to effectively communicate with the patient and their family (while respecting confidentiality)

- The results of the assessment.
- The risks and benefits of the proposed treatment plan, including possible side effects of psychotropic medications.
- Alternatives (if any) to proposed treatment plan.
- Education concerning the disorder, its prognosis, and prevention strategies.

Professionalism

The concept of professionalism has drawn a great deal of recent attention for its intangible, difficult-to-define quality (Kuczewski 2001; Misch 2002). One is tempted to resort to the words of Supreme Court Justice Potter Stewart from his famous 1964 opinion, wherein he wrote, "I know it when I see it." This definition is, of course, inadequate when making important decisions about a trainee's future abilities as a clinician and does an injustice to the qualities inherent in a professional. Abdicating the responsibility of instilling professional values in trainees is likewise a betrayal of the public trust, whose vested interests in training competent physicians has been an important stimulus toward competency-based education. Defining exactly what attitudes, skills, and behaviors contribute to professionalism, though, will be an ongoing challenge for psychiatry training programs in the coming decade.

The ACGME has decided that "[r]esidents must demonstrate a commitment to carrying out professional responsibilities, adherence to ethical principles, and sensitivity to a diverse patient population." Competency in this area will be established by residents' ability to

- Demonstrate respect, compassion, and integrity; a responsiveness to the needs of patients and society that supercedes self-interest; accountability to patients, society, and the profession; and a commitment to excellence and ongoing professional development.
- Demonstrate a commitment to ethical principles pertaining to provision or withholding of clinical care, confidentiality of patient information, informed consent, and business practices.
- Demonstrate sensitivity and responsiveness to patients' culture, age, gender, and disabilities.

An outline of the psychiatry-specific components of the Professionalism General Competency, as developed by Drs. Beresin, Davis, Herman, and Russell, follows.

1. The resident shall demonstrate responsibility for his or her patients' care. This responsibility includes
   - Responding to patients' communications.
   - Using the medical record for appropriate documentation of the course of illness and its treatment, providing coverage if unavailable (e.g., out of town, on vacation), and coordinating care with other members of the medical and/or multidisciplinary team.
   - Providing for appropriate transfer or referral if necessary.

2. The resident will respond to communication from patients and health professionals in a timely manner. If unavailable, the resident will establish and communicate backup arrangements. The resident communicates clearly to patients and families about how to seek emergent and urgent care when necessary.

3. The resident shall demonstrate ethical behavior, as defined in the American Psychiatric Association's *Principles of Medical Ethics With Annotations Specially Applicable to Psychiatry*.
4. The resident shall demonstrate respect for culturally diverse patients and colleagues as persons, including their cultural identity (as influenced by age, gender, race, ethnicity, socioeconomic status, religion/spirituality, sexual orientation, country of origin, acculturation, language, and disabilities, among other factors).
5. The resident ensures continuity of care for patients and when it is appropriate to terminate care, does so appropriately, and does not "abandon" patients.

Systems-Based Practice

Systems-based practice has been defined as "understanding, accessing, and utilizing the resources, providers, and systems necessary to provide optimum care while collaborating with other members of the healthcare team to assist patients in dealing effectively with complex systems and to improve systematic processes of care" (Itani 2002). From the perspective of the ACGME Outcome Project, "Residents must demonstrate an awareness of and responsiveness to the larger context and system of healthcare and the ability to effectively call on system resources to provide care that is of optimal value." To do so, residents will need to

- Understand how their patient care and other professional practices affect other healthcare professionals, the healthcare organization, and the larger society and how these elements of the system affect their own practice.
- Know how types of medical practice and delivery systems differ from one another, including methods of controlling healthcare costs and allocating resources.
- Practice cost-effective healthcare and resource allocation that does not compromise quality of care.
- Advocate for quality patient care and assist patients in dealing with system complexities.
- Know how to partner with healthcare managers and healthcare providers to assess, coordinate, and improve healthcare and know how these activities can affect system performance.

An outline of the psychiatry-specific components of the Systems-Based Practice General Competency, as developed by Drs. Beresin, Davis, Herman, and Russell, follows.

1. The resident shall be able to articulate the <u>basic concepts</u> of systems theory and of how it is used in psychiatry. The resident should have a working knowledge of the diverse systems involved in treating adults, children, and adolescents from culturally diverse backgrounds and understand how to use the systems as part of a comprehensive system of care, in general, and as part of a comprehensive, individualized treatment plan.

2. In the community system, the resident shall have

   - Knowledge of the resources available both publicly and privately for the treatment of psychiatric/behavioral problems and aimed at improving and enhancing the patient's quality of life.
   - Knowledge of the legal aspects of mental health as they impact patients with psychiatric problems (and their families).

3. The resident shall demonstrate knowledge of and interact with managed behavioral health systems. This shall include

   - Participating in utilization review communications and advocating for quality patient care.
   - Educating patients and families concerning such systems of care.

4. The resident shall demonstrate knowledge of community systems of care and assist patients to access appropriate psychiatric care and other mental health support services. This requires a knowledge of psychiatric treatment settings in the community that include ambulatory, consulting, inpatient, partial hospital, substance abuse, halfway houses, nursing homes, and hospices. The resident should demonstrate ability to integrate the care of patients across such settings. The entire process should be accomplished in a culturally sensitive and responsive manner.

References

Caraccio C, Wolfsthal SD, Englander R, et al: Shifting paradigms: from Flexner to competencies. Acad Med 77(5): 361–367, 2002

Epstein RM, Hundert EM: Defining and assessing professional competence. JAMA 287(2):226–235, 2002

Itani K: A positive approach to core competencies and benchmarks for graduate medical education. Am J Surg 184(3): 196–203, 2002

Kuczewski MG: Developing competency in professionalism: the potential and the pitfalls. ACGME Bulletin, October 2001, pp 3–6

Misch DA: Evaluating physicians' professionalism and humanism: the case for humanism "connoisseurs." Acad Med 77(6):489–495, 2002

Swing S: A report of the activities of the RRC Outcome Project Think Tank. ACGME Bulletin, November 2002, p 7

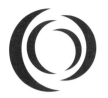

6

Defining Knowledge, Skills, and Attitudes to Be Taught for Each Psychotherapy Competency

This chapter includes lists of Sample Competencies for each of the Psychotherapy Competencies endorsed by the Psychiatry RRC. These Sample Competencies were developed by work groups of the American Association of Directors of Psychiatric Residency Training (AADPRT) Task Force on Competency. Input to the Task Forces was provided by residency training directors, psychotherapy experts from the AADPRT and the American Psychiatric Association's (APA) Commission on Psychotherapy by Psychiatrists, and residents.

The lists probably include more competency components for each psychotherapy competency than can realistically be taught and evaluated by any single residency program. Few programs will have the clinical material or the faculty resources to teach and evaluate every one of the component parts of the five psychotherapy competencies. These Sample Competencies are meant to guide residency program directors as each program director delineates the specific knowledge, skills, and attitudes that will be taught and then assessed within his or her own residency program for the five psychotherapy competencies. Each residency program's specific choices, from among the many possible sets of knowledge, skills, and attitudes, ought to reflect

the program's unique commitment to teaching psychotherapy. Each residency program's psychotherapy curriculum, didactic and clinical, similarly should represent the residency program's vision for optimal psychotherapy education and its commitment to producing residents competent in a set of core psychotherapy knowledge, skills, and attitudes. The persons listed as authors for each of the psychotherapy competencies lists spent considerable time and energy to produce these lists. The psychiatry education field can expect that these lists might be revised in a few years, as more residency programs gain experience in implementing the five Psychotherapy Competencies.

Brief Therapy Competencies[1]

Knowledge

1. The resident will demonstrate understanding of the spectrum of theoretical models and clinical concepts of brief therapy.
2. The resident will demonstrate understanding of the use of a focus and time limit as therapeutic tools.

---

[1]Authors: John Markowitz, M.D., Lisa Mellman, M.D., Eugene Beresin, M.D., David Goldberg, M.D., and Sandra DeJong, M.D. Revised November 21, 2001.

3. The resident will demonstrate understanding of the course of brief therapy, including phases of the treatment.
4. The resident will demonstrate understanding of indications and contraindications for brief therapy.
5. The resident will demonstrate understanding of the use of brief therapy in the overall treatment needs of the patient.
6. The resident will demonstrate understanding that continued education in brief therapy is necessary for further skill development.

Skills

1. The resident will be able to select suitable patients for the particular model chosen for brief therapy.
2. The resident will be able to establish and maintain a therapeutic alliance.
3. The resident will be able to establish and adhere to a time limit.
4. The resident will be able to establish and adhere to a focus.
5. The resident will be able to utilize at least one well-defined model of brief therapy.
6. The resident will be able to educate the patient about the goals, objectives, and time frame of brief therapy.
7. The resident will be able to recognize and identify affects in the patient and himself or herself.
8. The resident will be able to develop a formulation using the brief therapy model selected.
9. The resident will be able to seek appropriate consultation and/or referral for specialized treatment.

Attitudes

1. The resident will be empathic, respectful, curious, open, nonjudgmental, collaborative, and able to tolerate ambiguity and display confidence in the efficacy of brief therapy.
2. The resident will be sensitive to the sociocultural, socioeconomic, and educational issues that arise in the therapeutic relationship.
3. The resident will be open to review of audio- or videotapes or direct observations of treatment sessions.

Cognitive Behavioral Therapy Competencies[2]

Knowledge

1. The resident will demonstrate understanding of the basic principles of the cognitive model, including the relationship of thoughts to emotion, behavior, and physiology; the concept of automatic thoughts and cognitive distortions; the common cognitive errors; and the significance and origin of core beliefs and relationship of schemas to dysfunctional thoughts and assumptions, behavioral strategies, and psychopathology.
2. The resident will demonstrate understanding of the cognitive formulations for the psychiatric conditions for which cognitive therapy is indicated.
3. The resident will demonstrate understanding of the indications and contraindications for cognitive therapy.
4. The resident will demonstrate understanding of the basic rationale for structuring a cognitive therapy session, and the focus on active, collaborative problem solving.
5. The resident will demonstrate understanding of the basic principles of psychoeducation and skills training during therapy and, when termination approaches, for relapse prevention.
6. The resident will demonstrate understanding of the basic principles underlying the use of behavioral techniques, including activity scheduling, exposure and response prevention, relaxation training, graded task assignment, and exposure hierarchies/systematic desensitization.
7. The resident will demonstrate understanding of the basic principles underlying the use of cognitive techniques, including identifying automatic thoughts, cognitive restructuring, problem solving, advantage/disadvantage analyses, examining the evidence, thought recording, and modification of core beliefs.
8. The resident will demonstrate understanding of the ways in which rating scales are an integral part of cognitive behavioral therapy.
9. The resident will demonstrate understanding that continued education in cognitive behavioral therapy is necessary for further skill development.

---

[2]Authors: Jesse Wright, M.D., Donna Sudak, M.D., Lisa Mellman, M.D., David Goldberg, M.D., Eugene Beresin, M.D., Carol Bernstein, M.D., and Michele Pato, M.D. Revised November 21, 2001.

Skills

1. The resident will be able to elicit data and conceptualize patients using the cognitive conceptualization framework.
2. The resident will be able to establish and maintain a therapeutic alliance.
3. The resident will be able to educate the patient about the cognitive model, including the centrality of core beliefs/schemas, and the responsibilities of the patient in actively engaging in treatment.
4. The resident will be able to educate the patient about the core beliefs/schemas most relevant to the presenting problem and help him or her understand the basic origin of these beliefs.
5. The resident will be able to structure and focus the therapy sessions, including collaboratively setting the agenda, bridging from the previous session, reviewing homework and assigning appropriate new homework, working on key problems, summarizing and closing the session, and eliciting and responding to feedback.
6. The resident will be able to utilize activity scheduling and graded task assignment to teach the patient to monitor behavior and to increase patient engagement in desirable mastery and pleasure behaviors.
7. The resident will be able to utilize relaxation techniques, exposure and response prevention, and graded exposure to feared situations.
8. The resident will be able to employ the dysfunctional thought record and measure the impact this has on mood and behavior.
9. The resident will be able to recognize and identify affects in the patient and himself or herself.
10. The resident will be able to effectively plan termination with patients, employing booster sessions as indicated and teaching relapse prevention techniques.
11. The resident will be able to write a cognitive behavioral formulation.
12. The resident will seek appropriate consultation and/or referral for specialized treatment.

Attitudes

1. The resident will be empathic, respectful, curious, open, nonjudgmental, collaborative, and able to tolerate ambiguity and display confidence in the efficacy of cognitive behavioral therapy.
2. The resident will be sensitive to the sociocultural, socioeconomic, and educational issues that arise in the therapeutic relationship.
3. The resident will be open to review of audio- or videotapes or direct observations of treatment sessions.

Psychodynamic Psychotherapy Competencies[3]

Knowledge

1. The resident will demonstrate understanding of the spectrum of theoretical models of psychodynamic psychotherapy.
2. The resident will demonstrate understanding of the clinical psychodynamic psychotherapy concepts of the unconscious, defense and resistance, and transference and countertransference.
3. The resident will demonstrate understanding that symptoms, behaviors, and motivations often have multiple and complex meanings that may not be readily apparent.
4. The resident will demonstrate understanding of the influence of development through the life cycle on thoughts, feelings, and behavior.
5. The resident will demonstrate understanding of the indications and contraindications for the psychiatric disorders and problems treated by psychodynamic psychotherapy.
6. The resident will demonstrate understanding that continued education in psychodynamic psychotherapy is necessary for further skill development.

Skills

1. The resident will be able to evaluate the capacity of the patient to engage in and utilize psychodynamic psychotherapy.

---

[3]Authors: Lisa Mellman, M.D., David Goldberg, M.D., Eugene Beresin, M.D., Elizabeth Auchincloss, M.D., William Sledge, M.D., and Andres Sciolla, M.D. Revised November 21, 2001.

2. The resident will be able to display effective interpersonal skills in building and maintaining a collaborative therapeutic alliance that promotes self-reflection and inquiry into the patient's inner life.
3. The resident will be able to establish treatment goals with the patient.
4. The resident will able to establish a treatment frame with the patient.
5. The resident will be able to engage the patient in exploring his or her history of experiences, sociocultural influences, relationship patterns, coping mechanisms, fears, traumas and losses, and hopes and wishes in order to understand the presenting problems.
6. The resident will able to effectively listen to the patient to understand nuance, meanings, and indirect communications.
7. The resident will able to recognize and identify affects in the patient and himself or herself.
8. The resident will be able to recognize, utilize, and manage aspects of transference and countertransference, defense, and resistance in the course of treatment.
9. The resident will be able to utilize self-reflection to learn about his or her own responses to patients to further the goals of treatment.
10. The resident will be able to utilize clarification and confrontation.
11. The resident will be able to utilize interpretation to manage transference/countertransference that impedes or disrupts the therapeutic process.
12. The resident will be able to manage and understand the meanings of termination.
13. The resident will be able to write a psychodynamic formulation.
14. The resident will be to seek appropriate consultation and/or referral for specialized treatment.

Attitudes

1. The resident will be empathic, respectful, curious, open, nonjudgmental, collaborative, and able to tolerate ambiguity and display confidence in the efficacy of psychodynamic psychotherapy.
2. The resident will be sensitive to sociocultural, socioeconomic, and educational issues that arise in the therapeutic relationship.

3. The resident will be open to audio- or videotapes or direct observations of treatment sessions.

Psychotherapy Combined With Psychopharmacology Competencies[4]

Knowledge

1. The resident will demonstrate knowledge of the diagnoses and clinical conditions that warrant consideration of psychopharmacologic treatment in addition to psychotherapy, and psychotherapy in addition to psychopharmacology.
2. The resident will demonstrate knowledge of different methods of combining psychotherapy and psychopharmacology.
3. The resident will demonstrate knowledge of the specific indications for a recommendation of psychotherapy and psychopharmacology and the rationale for the type of psychotherapy and medication recommended.
4. The resident will demonstrate knowledge of potential synergies and/or antagonisms in combining psychotherapy and psychopharmacology.
5. The resident will demonstrate knowledge that taking medication may have multiple psychological and sociocultural meanings to a patient.
6. The resident will demonstrate knowledge of the background, education, and training of other mental health professionals who may provide psychotherapy in a combined treatment.
7. The resident will demonstrate understanding that continued education in combined psychotherapy and psychopharmacology is necessary for further skill development.

Skills

1. The resident will be able to gather sufficient clinical information to assess the need for, recommend, and implement combined (sequential or simultaneous) psychotherapy and psychopharmacology.
2. The resident will be able to form an active alliance with the patient that facilitates adherence to combined psychotherapy and psychopharmacology.

---

[4]Authors: John Sargent, M.D., Paul Mohl, M.D., Bernie Beitman, M.D., Eugene Beresin, M.D., Lisa Mellman, M.D., and Jessica Roberts, M.D. Revised November 21, 2001.

3. The resident will be able to monitor the patient's condition and modify the psychotherapeutic or psychopharmacologic approach when necessary.
4. The resident will be able to appreciate and assess the importance of timing of psychotherapeutic and psychopharmacologic interventions.
5. The resident will be able to understand the influences of other factors on combined psychotherapy and psychopharmacology, such as conscious and unconscious aspects of the doctor-patient relationship, placebo effects, and concurrent medical conditions.
6. The resident will be able to recognize and identify affects in the patient and himself or herself.
7. The resident will be able to use psychotherapeutic techniques to diminish resistance to and facilitate use of medication when appropriate.
8. The resident will be able to recognize the potential beneficial and/or detrimental effects of medication use in a psychotherapeutic treatment.
9. The resident will be able to understand and explore the psychological and sociocultural meaning to a patient of taking medication.
10. The resident will be able to collaborate effectively with nonpsychiatric psychotherapists and respond to conflicts and problems in the three-person treatment.

Attitudes

1. The resident will be empathic, respectful, curious, open, nonjudgmental, collaborative, and able to tolerate ambiguity and display confidence in the efficacy of combined psychotherapy and psychopharmacology.
2. The resident will be sensitive to the sociocultural, socioeconomic, and educational issues and belief systems that arise in the therapeutic setting.
3. The resident will understand that treatment is integrated such that the individual components of combined psychotherapy and psychopharmacology constitute the whole treatment and are not divisible into independent parts.
4. The resident will be open to audio- or videotapes or direct observations of treatment sessions.

Supportive Therapy Competencies[5]

Knowledge

1. The resident will demonstrate knowledge that the principal objectives of supportive therapy are to maintain or improve the patient's self-esteem, minimize or prevent recurrence of symptoms, and maximize the patient's adaptive capacities.
2. The resident will demonstrate understanding that the practice of supportive therapy is commonly utilized in many therapeutic encounters.
3. The resident will demonstrate knowledge that the patient-therapist relationship is of paramount importance.
4. The resident will demonstrate knowledge of indications and contraindications for supportive therapy.
5. The resident will demonstrate understanding that continued education in supportive therapy is necessary for further skill development.

Skills

1. The resident will be able to establish and maintain a therapeutic alliance.
2. The resident will be able to establish treatment goals.
3. The resident will be able to interact in a direct and nonthreatening manner.
4. The resident will be able to be responsive to the patient and give feedback and advice when appropriate.
5. The resident will be able to demonstrate the ability to understand the patient as a unique individual within his or her family, sociocultural, and community structure.
6. The resident will be able to determine which interventions are in the best interest of the patient and exercise caution about basing interventions on his or her own beliefs and values.
7. The resident will be able to recognize and identify affects in the patient and himself or herself.
8. The resident will be able to confront in a collaborative manner behaviors that are dangerous or damaging to the patient.

[5]Authors: Henry Pinsker, M.D., Lisa Mellman, M.D., Eugene Beresin, M.D., David Goldberg, M.D., Donald Misch, M.D., and Lee Ascherman, M.D. Revised November 21, 2001.

9. The resident will be able to provide reassurance to reduce symptoms, improve morale and adaptation, and prevent relapse.

10. The resident will be able to support, promote, and recognize the patient's ability to achieve goals that will promote his or her well-being.

11. The resident will be able to provide strategies to manage problems with affect regulation, thought disorders, and impaired reality testing.

12. The resident will be able to provide education and advice about the patient's psychiatric condition, treatment, and adaptation while being sensitive to specific community systems of care and sociocultural issues.

13. The resident will be able to demonstrate that, in the care of patients with chronic disorders, attention should be directed to adaptive skills, relationships, morale, and potential sources of anxiety or worry.

14. The resident will be able to assist the patient in developing skills for self-assessment.

15. The resident will be able to seek appropriate consultation and/or referral for specialized treatment.

Attitudes

1. The resident will be empathic, respectful, curious, open, nonjudgmental, collaborative, and able to tolerate ambiguity and display confidence in the efficacy of supportive therapy.

2. The resident will be sensitive to sociocultural, socioeconomic, and educational issues that arise in the therapeutic relationship.

3. The resident will be open to audio- or videotapes or direct observations of treatment sessions.

7

Incorporating the General and Psychotherapy Competencies in the Residency Program Curriculum

The recommended list of specific knowledge, skills, and attitudes to be taught and assessed for the six General Competencies and five Psychotherapy Competencies is quite lengthy. The Accreditation Council for Graduate Medical Education (ACGME) Outcome Project document refers to 28 different elements within the six General Competencies. The Psychiatry-Specific Competencies list 167 different components within the six General Competencies. The American Association of Directors of Psychiatric Residency Training (AADPRT) Task Force on Competency, in its November 21, 2001, Sample Psychotherapy Competencies document, designates 109 different knowledge, skills, and attitudes elements within the five Psychotherapy Competencies. Program directors will likely differ considerably on how meticulously they wish to document these 304 elements and where and when in the overall curriculum each of them might be taught and evaluated. Many program directors will choose to document competency achievement more generally, for only the six General Competencies and five Psychotherapy Competencies, but not for each of the 304 different components within those larger competency categories.

Whichever way a program director decides to tackle this challenge, he or she would first need to determine where within the clinical and didactic curriculum each competency component would be best taught. Next, the program director would need to determine additional curricular elements in which that given competency component could be taught, to augment the teaching within the existing curriculum. Said differently, the program director should create a list of curricular elements in which each competency will be taught and evaluated. Factors to be considered in deciding how best to teach a given competency include the following:

- Optimal postgraduate year in which the didactic or clinical teaching should occur. How does achieving competency in one area affect a resident's ability to develop additional competencies in other areas? Those competency components required as building blocks for other competency components should be taught earlier in the curriculum, allowing optimal sequencing and mastery development.
- Optimal intensity of supervision required to ensure patient safety while the resident develops competence.
- Estimated length of time to obtain the specific knowledge, skills, or attitudes requisite to develop any given

competency and estimated volume of clinical experience that is likely to be needed to demonstrate competence. Those competency components that require either many different patient encounters or long-term relationships with patients will need to be integrated early into the curriculum to allow adequate time for competency development.

- Best assessment method for any given competency.

Once the program director has decided where to teach each competency, including some or all of its component parts, then he or she must specify how each competency will be assessed. Just as each competency will ideally be taught in multiple settings through a variety of teaching methods, each competency will also, ideally, be assessed in multiple settings through a variety of assessment methods. The ACGME, using its Toolbox of Assessment Methods© (see appendix to Chapter 4 in this book), has suggested best methods for evaluating each of the six General Competencies. These best-method suggestions differ for the six General Competencies because the knowledge, skills, and attitudes to be taught and measured for the six General Competencies differ relatively dramatically. The ACGME's assessment recommendations are intended to serve as guides for residency program directors, not as proscriptions or requirements. The ACGME recommendations follow.

Patient Care

- Standardized patient
- Objective-structured clinical examination (OSCE)
- Patient survey
- Chart review

Medical Knowledge

- Examination—multiple choice questions
- Oral examination
- Chart review

Practice-Based Learning and Improvement

- Examination—multiple choice questions
- Oral examination
- Chart review
- 360-degree global ratings
- Portfolios

Interpersonal and Communication Skills

- Standardized patient
- OSCE
- Patient survey

Professionalism

- OSCE
- 360-degree global ratings
- Patient survey

Systems-Based Practice

- 360-degree global ratings
- Examination—multiple choice questions
- Patient survey
- Chart review

Program directors would be well advised to create an implementation grid or table that lists all of the competencies, including when, where, and how each would be taught and when, where, and how each would be evaluated. An example of an implementation grid for the overarching Cognitive Behavioral Psychotherapy (CBT) Competency might look something like the one on the opposite page.

By creating such a grid, program directors will easily recognize areas in which improvement is required. Specifically, program directors will be able to identify didactic or clinical components of the residency program that need to be expanded or developed to fill educational gaps. Program directors will also be able to identify evaluation deficiencies that need to be corrected and can then determine how they wish to expand or develop assessment methods to fill evaluation gaps.

In the near future, the ACGME and Residency Review Committee (RRC) will expect evaluation methods to extend beyond the typical written clinical evaluation to include more comprehensive evaluation methods such as nursing evaluations of resident performance, patient satisfaction surveys, and peer review. Scrutinizing a residency program's implementation grid should help program directors identify areas that require immediate improvement and those for which long-range planning might best accommodate these more complicated and comprehensive evaluation methods. Filling in every box on such an implementation grid would likely be impossible for any residency program director. Creating such a grid, rather, will serve as a reminder to residency pro-

CBT Competency	Teaching method	Evaluation method
	Didactic: PGY-II 12 sessions CBT seminar	Seminar evaluation form, with specific notation of attendance and participation
	Clinical: PGY-III three to five patients seen in outpatient clinics	Clinical evaluations (completed every 6 months for each rotation)
		Psychotherapy evaluations (completed every 6 months by two individual supervisors)
		Note: A resident must receive at least four evaluations that rank the resident as competent, without any ranking the resident as not yet competent, to be granted competency status for CBT.
	Other	PRITE: Review performance on relevant exam questions
		Mock Board examination: Review performance on relevant portions of the Mock Board examination

Note.   PRITE=Psychiatry Resident In-Training Examination.

gram directors that they need not reinvent the wheel for teaching and evaluating each and every general or psychotherapy competency. Program directors are encouraged to borrow good ideas from other psychiatry program directors or from other specialty program directors at their home institutions. At some future date, the ACGME anticipates publishing "best practices" so that program directors might supplement areas of deficiency within their own program with borrowed ideas from other programs.

Creating such an implementation grid in and of itself cannot prove that any given resident graduating from a residency program has attained all of the General and Psychotherapy Competencies. The grid, however, provides the first step in demonstrating that it would be possible for all residents graduating from a residency program to be taught and to attain all the competencies.

The next step in truly incorporating the competencies into the residency program would be to relate that individual resident's outcomes (evaluations of performance) back to his or her anticipated future didactic and clinical experiences and make modifications, where indicated, to ensure further competency development. The final incorporation step would be to relate group outcomes back to the training program's overall effectiveness at providing the didactic and clinical experiences that are necessary to produce residents who are competent to practice medicine in the current and ever-changing healthcare environment. These group outcomes could include overall evaluations of residents' performance during residency training and after graduation. Graduates' pass rates on Parts I and II of the American Board of Psychiatry and Neurology examination could provide some postresidency training data.

8

Program Director's To-Do List

This chapter is designed to be used as a practical checklist by residency program directors. The checklist will, it is hoped, help program directors assess their progress in incorporating and implementing the six General Competencies and the five Psychotherapy Competencies and help mechanize program directors' future planning for further incorporating and implementing the competencies into their residency programs. The to-do list should also help program directors prepare for their next Residency Review Committee (RRC) site visit.

For each item on the checklist, the program director should indicate whether that item has been **completed,** is **started and in progress** of being completed, or **not yet started.**

For each **completed** item, the program director should document the following:

- *When* and *how* the item was completed
- When it would need to be *repeated*

For each **started and in progress** item, the program director should document the following:

- The *next step*
- *Who is responsible* for the next step
- *Estimated date of completion* of the next step

For each **not yet started** item, the program director should document the following:

- The *next step*
- *Who is responsible* for the next step
- *Estimated date of completion* of the next step

Program Director's To-Do List

1. **Review clinical curriculum.**		
Completed _____	**Started and in progress** _____	**Not yet started** _____

❑ Cross-check to match with Program Requirements.

❑ Ensure that the clinical curriculum is designed to satisfy each time-based requirement. Develop a tracking mechanism for documenting/tracking the time-based requirements. (See sample time-based requirement checklist in Appendix C in this book.)

❑ Establish the program's optimal clinical learning environment(s) for each of the six General Competencies and five Psychotherapy Competencies. Detail this in writing, with site-specific descriptions.

❑ Determine if current educational opportunities within the program are sufficient to ensure each graduate's competency in the six General Competencies and five Psychotherapy Competencies mandated by the Accreditation Council for Graduate Medical Education (ACGME) and Psychiatry Residency Review Committee (RRC). Augment or change clinical rotations where improvement is needed.

❑ Use outcome data (e.g., PRITE [Psychiatry Resident In-Training Examination] scores, objective structured clinical examinations [OSCEs], Mock Board examinations, graduates' follow-up surveys, patient satisfaction surveys) to shape the program's clinical curriculum, over time, to ensure that individuals are attaining satisfactory levels of competence.

2. **Review didactic curriculum.**		
Completed _____	**Started and in progress** _____	**Not yet started** _____

❑ Cross-check to match with Program Requirements.

❑ Ensure that the didactic curriculum covers every specified content area from the Program Requirements.

❑ Establish the program's optimal didactic learning experiences for each of the six General Competencies and five Psychotherapy Competencies.

❑ Determine if current educational opportunities within the program are sufficient to ensure each graduate's competency in the six General Competencies and five Psychotherapy Competencies. Augment or change didactic schedules where improvement is needed.

❑ Use outcome data (e.g., PRITE scores, OSCEs, Mock Board examinations, graduates' follow-up surveys, patient satisfaction surveys) to shape the program's didactic curriculum, over time, to ensure that individuals are attaining satisfactory levels of competence.

3. **Revise goals and objectives.**		
Completed ____	**Started and in progress** ____	**Not yet started** ____

❏ Ensure that the goals and objectives are written for each clinical rotation at every postgraduate year level. Ideally, the faculty supervisor or coordinator for each clinical rotation should develop the rotation goals and objectives, with guidance from the site residency director, the residency program director, and possibly the curriculum committee.

❏ Ensure that the goals and objectives include language that coordinates with the six General Competencies and five Psychotherapy Competencies.

If the goals and objectives are not yet written, they should be written to incorporate the six General Competencies and five Psychotherapy Competencies, where applicable. If the goals and objectives already exist, they should be reviewed to ensure that they incorporate the six General Competencies and five Psychotherapy Competencies, where applicable. Efforts should be made to accentuate the competencies in rotations where they are already being taught and to add them, if appropriate, to rotations where they are currently not being taught. For example, a rotation within a community hospital in which trainees must negotiate several payor types and follow-up options should be identified as a Systems-Based Practice learning opportunity and the objectives to be learned about Systems-Based Practice should be included in the written goals and objectives for that rotation. (Example goals and objectives are provided in Appendix H in this book.)

❏ Identify goals and objectives that need to be written or rewritten.

4. **Revise evaluation instruments and add assessment methods.**		
Completed ____	**Started and in progress** ____	**Not yet started** ____

❏ List evaluation instruments currently being used.

❏ Ensure that the instruments include language that coordinates with the six General Competencies and five Psychotherapy Competencies.

If they do not, modify the program's clinical rotation evaluation forms to include the six General Competencies to underscore the importance of these areas to trainees and faculty. (Sample evaluation forms are provided in Appendix A in this book.) This modification can best be accomplished through an evaluation subcommittee of the curriculum committee or an evaluation retreat. Modify the program's psychotherapy supervision evaluation forms to reflect the five Psychotherapy Competencies. (See Appendix B in this book for a sample evaluation form. For additional examples of evaluation forms, see the American Association of Directors of Psychiatric Residency Training [AADPRT] [www.aadprt.org] and Association for Academic Psychiatry [AAP] [www.academicpsychiatry.org] websites.)

❏ List or create an inventory of competency assessment measures that are already being used within the residency program.

Such measures are usually separate and apart from clinical rotations, but they may be a component of the larger training program. This inventory might include in-service examinations (e.g., PRITE), Mock Board examinations, OSCEs, standardized patient examinations, journal club presentations, or any other measures of educational or clinical accomplishment. Designate the competencies being assessed by each assessment measure. (See Appendix F in this book for a sample inventory form.)

❏ Using the ACGME Toolbox of Assessment Methods© for guidance, supplement the program's assessment system in those areas in which evaluation of the General Competencies and Psychotherapy Competencies is weak or inadequate.

The Toolbox of Assessment Methods is available in Chapter 4 of this book or from the ACGME at its website (www.acgme.org/outcome/assess/toolbox.asp).

❏ Consider developing an implementation grid or table to document all assessment methods used by the program, including clinical rotation evaluations and the inventory of other assessment measures described earlier.

Although this grid will not be able to prove any given resident's competency in any area, it will list, in a single document, all the ways any given resident's competence will be assessed. (See table of sample assessment methods in Appendix F to this book.)

5. Create residency competency tracking system.		
Completed ____	**Started and in progress** ____	**Not yet started** ____

❏ Determine how you currently track/document patient experiences for each resident.

Many residency programs have moved to a computerized or personal digital assistant–based means for documenting patient logs. Workshops at the AADPRT annual meeting often review options for such tracking systems, and this issue is frequently discussed among residency program directors on the AADPRT Listserv or website (www.aadprt.org).

❏ Determine how you currently track/document resident completion of timed program requirements for each resident.

Many residency program directors have adopted a similar one-page form to document the time-based requirements (see Appendix C in this book for an example).

❏ Determine how you currently track/document achievement of completion of the six General Competencies and five Psychotherapy Competencies for each resident.

This newest documentation requirement provides the greatest current challenge to residency program directors. A sample tracking form, which is still undergoing revision at Baylor College of Medicine, is included in Appendix E in this book. This form is being designed to be used midyear as part of the semiannual evaluation process for residents in postgraduate years II, III, and IV. A variety of assessment methods will be recorded as either supporting or not supporting a resident's competence for his or her level of training for a given competency being evaluated (marked as *yes* or *no* on the sample form). Once a resident has received at least six positive measures indicating competence for level of training without receiving any negative measures indicating failure to achieve competence, the resident will be marked as having achieved competency for that particular one of the six General or five Psychotherapy Competencies. Using this tracking document midyear will allow feedback from the semiannual evaluations to be available for the residency program's progressions committee to review. Most program directors must make decisions about reappointment at least 4 months prior to the start of the next academic year. Therefore, data from this midyear tracking document could be used to inform reappointment decisions. It is probably more important, at this phase of implementation of the Outcome Project, to use some specific mechanism, albeit incomplete, for trying to track individual residents' competency than to worry whether the mechanism is exactly perfect.

❏ Begin to collect, systemically, programmatic outcome data on the successes and difficulties of individual trainees at achieving competence in the required areas in order to identify areas of strength and weakness within the residency program's unique curriculum.

Reports from the program's progressions committee could provide such data on a regular and continual basis.

❏ Collect data on the postgraduation performance of the program's residents as an additional source of evidence that the overall assessment of resident competence at graduation was accurate.

Performance on Board Certification examinations is one such measure of postgraduation assessment.

❏ Regularly review outcome data for individual and group trainee performance within the program's curriculum committee in order to assess the program's achievements in providing competency-based educational success over time.

Reports from the program's progressions committee, as well as resident performance on written or oral in-service examinations, should be included in these reviews. Data collected on the postgraduation performance of the program's residents should also be included in the curriculum committee's program reviews.

---

6. Educate (and reeducate) faculty and residents.

Completed ____	Started and in progress ____	Not yet started ____

❏ Determine whether you have had any educational programs to teach faculty and residents about the competencies.
Resident and faculty orientation presentations, departmental grand rounds, faculty meetings, and institutional graduate medical education lectures or workshops are just a few examples of ways to provide regular education to faculty and residents about the importance of the six General Competencies and five Psychotherapy Competencies to residency education. These forums also provide an opportunity to help faculty and residents understand the critical role that each plays in implementing the competencies within the clinical and didactic curriculum in a meaningful way. Some faculty and resident teaching about the competencies should occur each year. Faculty will need to understand their obligation to complete clinical rotation and individual supervision evaluations that document residents' achievement of competency (or not). Faculty will need to agree to provide remedial clinical and didactic experiences for residents who have not yet achieved competency to the program director's and progression committee's satisfaction. Faculty and residents will need to agree to review residency program goals and objectives and residency program feedback with special attention to how well (or not) the clinical and didactic curriculum is teaching the six General Competencies and five Psychotherapy Competencies. The residency program director alone cannot create, on paper or in actuality, a residency program that effectively achieves a competency-based education for its residents. Faculty and residents must understand that they are critical players in guaranteeing effective implementation of a competency-based residency education program. In return, faculty and residents should be acknowledged and appreciated for the important contributions that they make to ensuring the residency program's compliance with the ACGME and Psychiatry RRC Program Requirements, especially those related to the competencies. In particular, the program director should document annually, in writing, to each faculty member's teaching file or as part of each faculty member's annual faculty review, the important and effective teaching contributions that the faculty member has made to the residency program's mission of educating and training competent psychiatrists.

---

7. Determine when next RRC site visit is scheduled to take place.

Completed ____	Started and in progress ____	Not yet started ____

❏ Review the residency program's most recent previously submitted Program Information Form (PIF) if you have not already done so.

❏ Review the last two RRC letters for the residency program if you have not already done so.

❏ Determine when the next scheduled institutional internal review of the residency program is and carefully prepare for the program's internal review.
Welcome the recommendations of the internal review as helpful guidance toward creating an educationally successful program in full compliance with the ACGME. Use the internal review as another means for educating residents and faculty about the importance of the six General Competencies and five Psychotherapy Competencies as they relate to residency program accreditation.

❏ Identify key areas that need improvement.

❏ Solicit faculty members and residents to assist in doing a more in-depth review of the identified problem areas.

❏ At least 6 months before the scheduled site visit, develop a specific plan to prepare for the site visit.
Decide early who will help and in what very specific ways each person will help. Develop a written preparation plan that includes a list of tasks and a matching list of individuals responsible for completing and documenting completion of the tasks. Share written preparation plan, including the timetable for the completion of all tasks, with advisory committee and/or curriculum committee and with the department chairman and his or her executive committee. Creating a specific preparation plan and sharing the plan with many invested others will help ensure a successful site visit. Ultimately, the preparation responsibility lies with you as program director. However, bearing responsibility for and doing all of the preparation by yourself are two very different things.

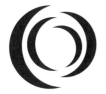

9

Rotation Coordinator's and Course Director's To-Do Lists

Faculty responsible for clinical rotations and didactic course work are crucial contributors to any program's success in transitioning to a competency-based curriculum. From implementation to evaluation to revision and improvement, these teaching physicians will be the "frontline troops" who make sure that curriculum changes are effective and lasting. This chapter offers two checklists for these faculty members to use to help them plan, accomplish, and revise their rotations and courses in order to realize the goal of a curriculum based on the six General Competencies and five Psychotherapy Competencies. The checklist identified for site or rotation coordinators is intended for any faculty member who is ac-

tively involved with clinical psychiatric education but particularly for those who are charged with the administration of educational efforts in a rotation format. The checklist for course directors is more focused on faculty members who are teaching in a didactic, seminar, group, colloquium, or other nonclinical setting. Clearly, there is some overlap, and the concepts are generally applicable across the curriculum. Likewise, the collaborative involvement of the residency director and departmental curriculum committee, at all steps of curriculum evolution, will be critical to produce a mechanical and philosophical shift of this magnitude in residency education.

Site or Rotation Coordinator's To-Do List

❑ Familiarize yourself with the specific knowledge, skills, and attitudes deemed necessary for trainees to demonstrate in the six General Competencies and five specific Psychotherapy Competencies of the Accreditation Council for Graduate Medical Education (ACGME) and Psychiatry Residency Review Committee (RRC).

❑ Work closely with the residency program director to understand the unique direction the program will take toward implementing a competency-based curriculum with adequate attention to the 11 competencies.

❑ Review the educational experiences offered by your rotation(s) and identify the optimum learning opportunities for each of the General and Specific competencies.

❑ Review (or create as necessary) the goals and objectives for each rotation hosted within your training site and identify the areas of competency-based education that already exist.

❑ Using the written goals and objectives, explicitly delineate the exact competency or competencies being taught or refined within each rotation and postgraduate year occurring at your site.

❑ Supplement, accentuate, or add language to the goals and objectives as possible to utilize every potential opportunity for education in the 11 competencies.

❑ Educate other involved faculty members at your site so that there is a general level of familiarity and sophistication with the ACGME and RRC competencies and a more specific understanding of the exact opportunities for developing these competencies offered by rotations within your institution or site.

❑ Reevaluate those assessment tools already used for the rotations at your site to ensure that there is adequate, explicit attention paid to objectively quantifying the six General Competencies and five Psychotherapy Competencies.

❑ Where there are opportunities for competency-based education but no evaluation tools being used within your site's rotations, identify the tools that might be used to help provide objective verification of trainees' competence.

❑ Work with the residency program director and site faculty to implement, update, and refine the identified assessment tools.

❑ Instruct faculty and residents on the accurate use of the evaluation tools.

❑ Begin using the assessment tools and collecting data on their ease of use, effectiveness, and accuracy over time.

❑ Establish procedures to remediate inadequate trainee or faculty performance in using the evaluation measures consistently and accurately.

❑ Working collaboratively with the residency program director and curriculum committee, develop remedial guidelines to be used when residents fail to achieve adequate competency milestones being tested within the evaluation process.

❑ Work with the residency program director and curriculum committee to revise and refine the evaluation tools as experience is developed.

❑ Gather feedback on the training and evaluation process from various stakeholders in the educational arena. Stakeholders might include faculty, residents, ancillary staff, clinic and hospital administrators, and even patients.

❑ As possible, monitor the residents' overall competency development during training and graduates' competence after completing training for the areas being taught and assessed within rotations at your site in order to ensure that the ultimate outcome of competency-based education, independent clinician competence, is being realized.

   As an example, ask the program director to provide you with residents' PRITE (Psychiatry Resident In-Training Examination) scores for the Child Psychiatry subcategory if you coordinate the PGY-II and PGY-III clinical rotations in child and adolescent psychiatry. Review these over time and adjust your clinical rotation design accordingly.

Didactic Course Director's To-Do List

❏ Familiarize yourself with the specific knowledge, skills, and attitudes deemed necessary for trainees to demonstrate in the six General Competencies and five specific Psychotherapy Competencies of the ACGME and Psychiatry RRC.

❏ Work closely with the residency program director to understand the unique direction the program will take to implementing a competency-based curriculum with adequate attention to the 11 areas.

❏ Review the educational experiences offered within your course and identify which of the general and specific areas of competence are emphasized within the substance of the sessions.

❏ Review the goals and objectives for the course, with attention to areas wherein the competencies might already be delineated.

❏ Modify the goals and objectives of the course such that each of the competencies included within the teaching is explicitly identified.

❏ Consider course modifications that could lead to new or enhanced educational opportunities in the various competencies, and implement these with the cooperation and guidance of the residency program director and curriculum committee.

❏ Review the evaluation system currently employed to monitor success in the educational goals and objectives for the course. Determine if there are areas of assessed competence already present within the evaluation system, and accentuate these within the course description, goals, and objectives.

❏ Consider either revising existing assessment tools or adding new ones to quantify learners' developing competency as a result of your educational intervention.
Use Chapter 7 of this text or the ACGME's Toolbox of Assessment Methods© (see appendix to Chapter 4) for guidance.

❏ Work with the residency program director and course faculty to implement the identified assessment tools.

❏ Instruct other faculty involved in teaching the course about the assessment method(s) being employed.

❏ Teach the residents about the purpose and correct usage of the assessment method(s) for the course. Repeat this for each new group of trainees.

❏ Begin using the assessment tools and collecting data on their ease of use, effectiveness, and accuracy over time.

❏ Establish procedures to remediate inadequate trainee or faculty performance in using the evaluation measures consistently and accurately.

❏ Working collaboratively with the residency program director and curriculum committee, develop remedial guidelines to be used when residents fail to adequately achieve competency milestones being tested within the course's evaluation process.

❏ Work with the residency program director and curriculum committee to revise and refine the evaluation tools as experience is developed.

❏ Gather feedback on the teaching and evaluation system from involved parties, particularly from co-teachers on the faculty and trainees who have completed the course.

❏ As possible, monitor the residents' overall competency development during training and the graduates' competence after completing training for the areas being taught and assessed within your course. This will ensure that the ultimate outcome of competency-based education, independent clinician competence, is being realized.
As an example, ask the residency program director for the PRITE scores for the Alcoholism and Substance Abuse subcategory if you coordinate and teach the residents' substance abuse courses. Alternatively, review summary performance feedback from Mock Board examinations regarding the residents' knowledge about alcoholism and substance abuse.

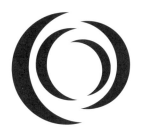

Part IV

Consideration of Other Interested Groups

Follow-Up With the ACGME, Psychiatry RRC, and ABPN

10

The Accreditation Council for Graduate Medical Education (ACGME) and the Psychiatry Residency Review Committee (RRC) have outlined how the Outcome Project will unfold over the next 10 years.

From July 2002 through June 2006, the ACGME and the Psychiatry RRC will review what is emerging from the field, provide citations related to the competencies that will have accreditation consequences, and revise Program Requirements. The American Association of Directors of Psychiatric Residency Training (AADPRT) plans to work proactively with the Psychiatry RRC to communicate feedback from the program directors in anticipation of the RRC's next revision of the Program Requirements. For site visits that take place through June 2006, program directors will be expected to provide evidence of learning in all six General Competencies and five Psychotherapy Competencies, to use progressively more dependable assessment tools, and to use evaluation data to assess effectiveness of resident learning.

From July 2006 through June 2011, the ACGME and all of the RRCs are expected to provide more specific guidance to programs, seek evidence that programs are using assessment for improvement, and share experiences across RRCs to identify best practices. For site visits that take place during this time period, program directors will be expected to provide evidence of learning in all six General Competencies and five Psychotherapy Competencies, to use assessments to improve programs overall, and to begin linking clinical quality indicators and patient surveys with educational outcomes.

Beyond 2011, the ACGME and all of the RRCs expect to identify benchmark programs, expand competencies to develop excellence models, and build knowledge about good graduate medical education.

At the institutional level, the Licensing Council on Medical Education (LCME) and the ACGME will have progressively higher expectations that university or institutional oversight of graduate medical education be more coordinated and comprehensive. These expectations will include clearer oversight and responsibility to ensure that all residency programs within their system are effectively incorporating the six General Competencies into education of residents. Specifically, institutional internal review processes will need to demonstrate a careful and thorough review process that assesses residency programs' compliance with implementing the six General Competencies.

Institutions that provide Continuing Medical Education (CME) will also need to develop ways to specify which of the six General Competencies are taught in any of its institutionally sponsored CME activities. As an example, Baylor College of Medicine's Office of Continuing Medical Education conducted a standardized review of its 2000–2001 CME activities, trying to classify which of the six General Competencies were taught in each CME activity. In doing so, the Office of CME hopes to catalogue its CME activities according to the six General Competencies and to identify which of the General Competencies were frequently taught or underrepresented in its most recent year of CME activities. The Office of CME may then choose to adjust future CME development to better address those General Competencies currently underrepresented in its CME offerings. The Office of CME is also trying to develop this standardized catalogue of its activities according to the General Competencies because it expects that practitioners will increasingly be expected to provide specialty boards with data demonstrating lifelong learning (CME) in all six General Competencies in order to maintain board certification status.

Most of the specialty boards anticipate making some adjustments in their initial board certification processes and in their recertification or maintenance of certification processes based on the General Competencies. Psychiatry residency program directors will need to stay abreast of the actions of the American Board of Psychiatry and Neurology (ABPN) regarding changes in both content and format of Part I and Part II of the ABPN examination and in the recertification examinations. In the near future, program directors will want to adjust the clinical skills exams given during residency training to better match the ABPN exam format changes. Program directors will also need to monitor how they advise residents to best prepare for their certification exams on the basis of the ABPN exam changes. To stay abreast of the ABPN's current status in incorporating the six General Competencies and five Psychotherapy Competencies into its certification and recertification processes, program directors should regularly review the ABPN website (www.abpn.com). Program directors might also consider reviewing a book recently published by the executive leadership of the ABPN, *Core Competencies for Psychiatric Practice: What Clinicians Need to Know* (Scheiber et al. 2003), which discusses exactly this topic.

Teaching and assessing resident competence in the General and Psychotherapy Competencies will provide ongoing challenges for residency program directors for years to come. According to Morreale and Backlund (1999), teaching and assessing these competencies in an effective manner will benefit residents, faculty, institutions in which we provide residency education, and patients. Six primary questions are posited as the fundamental questions that residency program directors will be expected to answer regarding the teaching and assessment methods that they have used in implementing the competencies fully into their residency training programs (Morreale and Backlund 1999):

- Who are you and why do you exist? (Mission)
- What do you want to accomplish? (Goals and objectives)

- What procedures will you use to determine if the goals and objectives have been met? (Assessment)
- What are the results of your assessment process? (Analysis)
- What changes will you make to your goals, objectives, outcomes, and processes on the basis of these results? (Application of results)
- What evidence do you have that this is a continuous cycle? (Continuous improvement)

Finally, the following list represents the top 10 characteristics of successful assessment programs, derived from the literature of accreditation associations, academic campuses, and professional associations (Morreale and Backlund 1999). Variations on this list might be useful for developing assessment programs within psychiatry residency education programs.

A successful assessment program

- Flows from an institution's mission, the department's mission and goals, course-specific goals, and student outcomes.
- Emerges from a conceptual framework for student learning.
- Is marked by faculty ownership, responsibility, and involvement.
- Has institution-wide support.
- Relies on the use of multiple methods and measures.
- Supports equal access and equity and honors diversity.
- Provides feedback to students, teachers, and the institution.
- Is cost-effective.
- Leads to desirable and valuable change and improvement.
- Includes a process for evaluating and assessing itself.

References

Morreale SP, Backlund PA: Assessment: Coming of Age. Washington, DC, National Communication Association, 1999. Available at: http://www.natcom.org/Instruction/assessment/Assessment/article99.htm. Accessed January 28, 2003

Scheiber SC, Kramer TAM, Adamowski SE: Core Competencies for Psychiatric Practice: What Clinicians Need to Know (A Report of the American Board of Psychiatry and Neurology, Inc.). Washington, DC, American Psychiatric Publishing, 2003

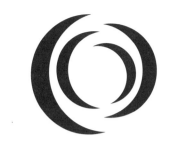

Appendixes

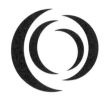

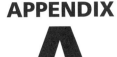

Anchored Clinical Rotation Evaluation Forms for Each Postgraduate Level of Training

Date reviewed by Residency Director: _____

PGY-I Clinical **Midpoint Feedback** and **Final End of Rotation Evaluation**

Resident's name: _____ Evaluator(s) (please print): _____

Rotation dates: ___/___/200__ to ___/___/200__ Rotation location: _____

A. Midpoint Feedback

Midpoint feedback provided on _____ _____ _____
   Date   *Faculty Signature(s)*   *Resident Signature*

B. Final End of Rotation Evaluation

Instructions for scoring: Rate the resident's skill in each of the categories 1–6 using the descriptions as a guide.
Darken bubbles ● with pen or pencil completely. Place emphasis on written comments at the end.

Please note: The gray column identifies competence at satisfactory levels. The two columns to its left denote unsatisfactory performance. The column to the immediate right of the gray column, identified with the symbol ⊕, denotes performance beyond satisfactory levels and is inclusive of the elements specified in the gray column. The extreme right column, identified with the symbol ⊕⊕, includes the *two* elements to its immediate left as well.

1. PATIENT CARE (THE APPLICATION OF KNOWLEDGE IN THE CLINICAL SETTING)

1A. Diagnostic Skills, Assessment and Evaluation	Takes cursory history, performs a minimal examination. Inaccurate data or major omissions in data gathered.	Some omissions, lacks supporting detail. Difficulty in interpreting or synthesizing data.	Obtains necessary historical data elements, includes essential positives and negatives. Can perform a reasonable mental status examination.	⊕ Gets extensive historical and examination information, seeks negative and positive findings in all fields. Effectively integrates data.	⊕⊕ Efficient, thorough data gathering. Accurate mental status examination with detailed cognitive exam. Performs assessment well beyond the training level.
	◯	◯	◯	◯	◯
1B. Ability to Develop Rapport and Therapeutic Alliance	Frequently unable to engage patient in interview. Tactless. Disrespectful.	Frequent difficulty engaging patient in interview and forming therapeutic alliance.	Makes patients comfortable enough to engage in evaluation process and treatment. Shows respect for patient.	⊕ Can engage patients well. Perceived as capable. Very respectful. Able to elicit cooperation even in awkward situations.	⊕⊕ Has patient's confidence. Works exceptionally well even with difficult patients. Maximizes patient adherence to treatment.
	◯	◯	◯	◯	◯
1C. Psychotherapy	Does not invite patient interaction beyond the evaluative phase.	Clueless about how to initiate therapy. Leaves it to others.	Empathic and able to set limits without being rigid. Can help with reality orientation. Can refer appropriately.	⊕ Can engage patients in psychotherapy. Identifies cognitive distortions and helps with reality orientation.	⊕⊕ Highly empathic. Psychotherapy skills far beyond the level expected.
	◯	◯	◯	◯	◯
1D. Pharmacotherapy	Does not titrate or taper. Makes several drug changes simultaneously. Oblivious to drug interactions.	Infrequently implements titration or tapering. Inconsistently identifies target symptoms. Poor appreciation of safety monitors, interactions.	Prescribes, titrates, and tapers standard medications at reasonable doses. Monitors and treats common side effects.	⊕ Prescribes, titrates, and tapers more than just the standard medications appropriately. Monitors and treats even some uncommon side effects.	⊕⊕ Proficient prescription of meds. Alert to side effects and drug-drug interactions far beyond the level expected.
	◯	◯	◯	◯	◯
1E. Treatment Planning	Difficulty understanding or formulating treatment options.	Needs prompting to identify elements of interdisciplinary treatment plan. Makes unrealistic treatment goals.	Satisfactory grasp of basic concepts and treatment options to synthesize a realistic, interdisciplinary treatment plan.	⊕ Expanded understanding of differential diagnosis and treatment options for treatment plan.	⊕⊕ Outstanding, covering continuity of care. Description clear and easy to follow. Maximizes outcome.
	◯	◯	◯	◯	◯
1F. Patient Communication and Education	No communication with patients or family. Patient often left in the dark, confused about treatment. No informed consent.	Family members, and sometimes patients, confused about treatment or instructions. Technical terms overused.	Consistently explains diagnoses, treatment, and risks and benefits in simple terms to patient and family. Considers patient preferences.	⊕ Explains and involves patient and family in decision process. Establishes therapeutic alliance even with volatile patients.	⊕⊕ Adapts speaking style to suit individual. Inspires confidence in even the most recalcitrant patients. Abilities well beyond those expected.
	◯	◯	◯	◯	◯

2. CLINICAL SCIENCE (FUND OF KNOWLEDGE, INCLUDING CONCEPTUAL THEORY AND SCIENTIFIC LITERATURE)

2A. Pharmacotherapy	Major deficiencies, little understanding of basic concepts. Confused about drug classes and indications. ○	Some deficiencies. Incomplete understanding of significant side effects and ways to monitor for safety. ○	Is aware of major medication classes, their indications. Has basic knowledge of management of common side effects. ○	⊕ Expanded understanding of therapeutic options, drug-drug interactions. Able to select by applying recent information. ○	⊕⊕ Mastery of drug effects and limits, current with state-of-the-art concepts. Comprehensive understanding of treatment options. ○
2B. Psychotherapy	Little knowledge beyond the fact that it involves listening and talking. ○	Marginal concept of types and indications. ○	Can name the different types of psychotherapy, their indications. Has some concept of background theories and application. ○	⊕ Familiar with different types of psychotherapies. Good grasp of theories, application, and indications for different types of psychotherapy. ○	⊕⊕ Excellent grasp of theories, application, and indications of different types of psychotherapy, especially CBT. Understands complex issues and interactions. ○
2C. Descriptive Psychiatry and Differential Diagnosis	Lacks background knowledge to understand common problems. Cannot interpret data. No prioritization. Likely to miss major disorder. Ignores factors contributing to pathology. ○	Some difficulty with interpretation of data and prioritization of issues. Sometimes ignores factors contributing to pathology. ○	Knows major DSM-IV categories and can come up with rational differential diagnoses. Familiar with relevant terminology and can define commonly used descriptive terms. ○	⊕ Can make DSM-IV and biopsychosocial formulations. Well versed with terminology. Very thorough with differential diagnosis. ○	⊕⊕ Excellent formulation. Synthesizes detailed differential diagnosis with appropriate prioritization of issues. Expanded grasp of terminology. ○

3. PRACTICE-BASED LEARNING AND IMPROVEMENT (RESIDENT'S ABILITY TO APPLY DAILY CLINICAL PRACTICE TO OWN LEARNING AND DEVELOPMENT)

	Makes same mistakes again and again. Oblivious of context. No appreciation of ethnic or cultural variations. ○	Needs frequent prompting to adjust. Slow to learn from previous mistakes. Minimal appreciation of ethnic or cultural variations. ○	Improves and adds to own development by learning from day-to-day clinical practice. Adapts to cultural backgrounds and work situations without undue assumptions. ○	⊕ Learns quickly from practice. Anticipates and adapts to different cultural backgrounds and work situations. Assimilates and applies relevant literature. ○	⊕⊕ Excellent learning from practice. Rapidly acquires, assimilates, and applies relevant literature. Recognizes and utilizes strengths and weaknesses of systems. ○

4. INTERPERSONAL AND COMMUNICATION SKILLS

4A. Working Relationships	Inappropriate, antagonistic, disruptive, arrogant, not respectful of peers or staff. ○	Inflexible, inconsiderate, frequently loses composure. ○	Good team member. Cordial to staff members; recognizes their contributions, knows when to consult others. Invites mutual respect. ○	⊕ Flexible, supportive, respectful, develops very good rapport with team. Recognizes the benefits and limits of others' skills. ○	⊕⊕ Poised, establishes tone of mutual respect. Invaluable team member. Recognizes talents within team. Brings out the best in others. ○
4B. Patient-Specific Skills	Avoids personal contact, tactless, inattentive to patients' feelings, impolite, arrogant, abusive. ○	Occasionally insensitive or inattentive, superficial. Reluctant to communicate with patients' families. ○	Empathic, listens attentively, develops rapport, adequate communication with patient and family. ○	⊕ Effective communication, perceived by patient and family as capable. Can handle some degree of volatility. ○	⊕⊕ Works directly with patient, inspiring confidence and compliance. Works exceptionally well even with difficult patients. ○
4C. Verbal Presentation	Inaccurate, major omissions, rambling, inappropriate comments. ○	Disorganized, unfocused, some omissions. Gives irrelevant or inaccurate information. ○	Complete, includes all basic information, with positives and relevant negatives. Follows usual format. ○	⊕ Well organized, thorough, precise. Effectively integrates data. Appreciates subtleties. Concise, comprehensive. ○	⊕⊕ Polished presentations, tailored to situation. Outstanding, discussion reflects thorough understanding of disorder and patient situation. ○

5. PROFESSIONALISM

5A. Management of Clinical Responsibility	Is often absent or late. Leaves patient care tasks unfinished. Lacks follow-up. Fails to plan. Misses changes in patient status. Delegates tasks inappropriately to reduce workload. Avoids assigned duty area. Fails to respond to paging. ○	Occasionally absent or late. Unavailable at times. Sometimes has others do what is assigned to resident. Erratic in planning and follow-up. Slow to see changes in patient status. Unreliable response to paging. ○	Satisfactory attendance, generally on time. Usually available when needed. Delegates appropriately. Adequate management plans and follow-up. Timely recognition of changes. Reliable response to paging. ○	⊕ Commendable attendance and punctuality. Always answers pages quickly. Thoughtful, detailed management plans. Regular follow-up, quick to see changes. ○	⊕⊕ Impeccably punctual, unswervingly diligent, immediately responsive. Anticipates needs. Seeks involvement in all parts of patient care and research. Eager for new skills. Insightful plans and follow-up. Suggests alternative. ○
5B. Documentation	Inaccurate data. Overdue. Misleading. Disorganized. Important portions missing. Rationale unclear. Change or progress unclear. Copied and pasted without editing. Typos abound. Poor grammar. Poses legal risk. ○	Occasional inaccuracies, poor organization, but rationale can be deciphered. Moderate risk potential. ○	Records generally coherent, timely, illustrate progression of treatment, include basic elements to satisfy billing, legal, and future patient care needs. ○	⊕ Notes timely, clearly show treatment rationale and progress, useful for reference. Medical record appreciated and handled as an integral part of patient care, risk management, and financial accountability. ○	⊕⊕ Well organized, focused, comprehensive. Records fully recognized as an important part of patient care and as a legal document. Always done completely and promptly, including dictation require-ments. ○
5C. Teaching	Makes no effort to convey information to students and poorly models seeking of information. ○	Answers students' ques-tion briefly if asked, but does not initiate any teaching. ○	Makes satisfactory effort to instruct and encourage students assigned. Rec-ognizes good teaching opportunities. ○	⊕ Consistently acknowl-edged as a teacher by students and other learners. ○	⊕⊕ Viewed by students and staff as *the* source of clinical and scientific data. Inspires learning and inde-pendent research. ○
5D. Ethical Decision Making, Honesty, Cultural Sensitivity	Does not apply acceptable moral standards to decision making. Often prejudiced. Attempts to camouflage errors. Does not share credit or accept blame. ○	Irregularly applies acceptable moral standards to decision making. Not always impartial. On occasion covers up mistakes and tends to take more credit than due. ○	Usually applies accept-able moral standards to personal and clinical decision making. Admits to errors. Generally able to give and take credit appropriately. ○	⊕ Quality decision making. Always applies sound moral standards to decision making. Admits to errors. Acknowledges equality of all people. ○	⊕⊕ Exceptional decision making, based on impec-cable moral standards. Respects human dignity, without bias. Recognizes responsibility to patient and to society. ○
5E. Personal Qualities	Does not seek information. Unreliable. Dawdles. Poor initiative. Leaves early and is inflexible. Overestimates ability. Unresponsive to criticism. Frequently looks sloppy. ○	Inefficient. Requires reminders to seek infor-mation. Often unwilling to do what is needed. Fails to seek supervision. Semiresponsive to criticism. Looks untidy at times. ○	Reads what is essential. Reliable follow-through. Effective time use. Works required time and gen-erally flexible, responsive to criticism. Seeks help when needed. Appears tidy and composed. ○	⊕ Eager to learn, seeks additional reading. Effi-cient, conscientious, and helpful. Seeks and responds to feedback. Clear view of limitations. Maintains a professional appearance. ○	⊕⊕ Highly motivated to expand knowledge and enhance productivity. Goes out of the way to help. Peers ask for advice. Maximizes personal strengths. Looks com-mendably professional. ○

6. SYSTEMS-BASED CARE (ABILITY TO ADAPT TO MENTAL HEALTH CARE FUNDING AND TO DIFFERENT TYPES OF DELIVERY SYSTEM)

	Lacks background knowl-edge to understand com-mon patient problems. Unable to work with elec-tronic records. Patient care plan insupportable. Oblivious to treatment algorithms. ○	Understands a few com-mon patient problems. Limited ability to work with electronic records. Patient care plan often insupportable. Marginally aware of treatment algorithms. ○	Cognizant of local patient population trends. Able to tailor patient care to resources available in system. Competent with relevant information tech-nology. Aware of local treatment algorithms. ○	⊕ Up-to-date with local patient population trends. Well aware of resources. Skillfully tailors patient care. Proficient with relevant information technology. Comfortable with local treatment algorithms. ○	⊕⊕ Fully aware of local patient trends, available resources. Mastery of information technology. Conforms to and improves upon consensus treatment algorithms. ○

Overall Rating	Not competent	Falls below expectations	Good, solid work	⊕ Exceeds expectations	⊕⊕ Far exceeds expectations
	◯	◯	◯	◯	◯

Assessment Methods (Select all that apply)	Direct observation	Records review	Discussion with resident	Videotape	Other_____
	◯	◯	◯	◯	◯

General comments:

Other areas of special talent:

Other areas where more work is needed (please elaborate on all *unsatisfactory* ratings [to the left of the gray column] and any significant discrepancies between overall rating and specific ratings):

I have reviewed this performance evaluation with the resident. _____ Date: _____
(Faculty Signature)

I have reviewed this evaluation with the faculty member. _____ Date: _____
(Resident Signature)

PLEASE RETURN TO LINDA ANDREWS, M.D., VIA INTER-INSTITUTIONAL MAIL BY _____   *Thank you* ☺

Date reviewed by Residency Director: _____

PGY-II Clinical **Midpoint Feedback** and **Final End of Rotation Evaluation**

Resident's name: _____ Evaluator(s) (please print): _____

Rotation dates: ___/___/200__ to ___/___/200__ Rotation location: _____

A. Midpoint Feedback

Midpoint feedback provided on _____ _____ _____

　　　　　　　　　　　　　　　　　Date　　　　　　　　　　*Faculty Signature(s)*　　　　　　　　　*Resident Signature*

B. Final End of Rotation Evaluation

Instructions for scoring: Rate the resident's skill in each of the categories 1–6 using the descriptions as a guide.
Darken bubbles ● with pen or pencil completely. Place emphasis on written comments at the end.

Please note: The gray column identifies competence at satisfactory levels. The two columns to its left denote unsatisfactory performance. The column to the immediate right of the gray column, identified with the symbol ⊕, denotes performance beyond satisfactory levels and is inclusive of the elements specified in the gray column. The extreme right column, identified with the symbol ⊕⊕, includes the *two* elements to its immediate left as well.

1. PATIENT CARE (THE APPLICATION OF KNOWLEDGE IN THE CLINICAL SETTING)

1A. Diagnostic Skills, Assessment and Evaluation	Cursory history, performs a minimal examination. Inaccurate data or major omissions in data gathered.	Some omissions, lacks supporting detail. Difficulty in interpreting or synthesizing data.	Obtains necessary historical data elements, includes essential positives and negatives. Can perform a reasonable mental status examination.	⊕ Gets extensive historical and examination information, seeks negative and positive findings in all fields. Effectively integrates data.	⊕⊕ Efficient, thorough data gathering. Accurate mental status examination with detailed cognitive exam. Performs assessment well beyond the training level.
	○	○	○	○	○
1B. Ability to Develop Rapport and Therapeutic Alliance	Frequently unable to engage patient in interview. Tactless. Disrespectful.	Frequent difficulty engaging patient in interview and forming therapeutic alliance.	Makes patients comfortable enough to engage in evaluation process and treatment. Shows respect for patient.	⊕ Can engage patients well. Perceived as capable. Very respectful. Able to elicit cooperation even in awkward situations.	⊕⊕ Has patient's confidence. Works exceptionally well even with difficult patients. Maximizes patient adherence to treatment.
	○	○	○	○	○
1C. Psychotherapy	Does not invite patient interaction beyond the evaluative phase.	Clueless about how to initiate therapy. Leaves it to others.	Empathic and able to set limits without being rigid. Can help with reality orientation. Can refer appropriately.	⊕ Can engage patients in psychotherapy. Identifies cognitive distortions and helps with reality orientation.	⊕⊕ Highly empathic. Psychotherapy skills far beyond the level expected.
	○	○	○	○	○
1D. Pharmacotherapy	Does not titrate or taper. Makes several drug changes simultaneously. Oblivious to drug interactions.	Infrequently implements titration or tapering. Inconsistently identifies target symptoms. Poor appreciation of safety monitors, interactions.	Prescribes, titrates, and tapers standard medications at reasonable doses. Monitors and treats common side effects.	⊕ Prescribes, titrates, and tapers more than just the standard medications appropriately. Monitors and treats even some uncommon side effects.	⊕⊕ Proficient prescription of meds. Alert to side effects and drug-drug interactions far beyond the level expected.
	○	○	○	○	○
1E. Treatment Planning	Difficulty understanding or formulating treatment options.	Needs prompting to identify elements of interdisciplinary treatment plan. Makes unrealistic treatment goals.	Satisfactory grasp of basic concepts and treatment options to synthesize a realistic, interdisciplinary treatment plan.	⊕ Expanded understanding of differential diagnosis and treatment options for treatment plan.	⊕⊕ Outstanding, covering continuity of care. Description clear and easy to follow. Maximizes outcome.
	○	○	○	○	○
1F. Patient Communication and Education	No communication with patients or family. Patient often left in the dark, confused about treatment. No informed consent.	Family members, and sometimes patients, confused about treatment or instructions. Technical terms overused.	Consistently explains diagnoses, treatment, and risks and benefits in simple terms to patient and family. Considers patient preferences.	⊕ Explains and involves patient and family in decision process. Establishes therapeutic alliance even with volatile patients.	⊕⊕ Adapts speaking style to suit individual. Inspires confidence in even the most recalcitrant patients. Abilities well beyond those expected.
	○	○	○	○	○

2. CLINICAL SCIENCE (FUND OF KNOWLEDGE, INCLUDING CONCEPTUAL THEORY AND SCIENTIFIC LITERATURE)

2A. Pharmacotherapy	Major deficiencies, little understanding of basic concepts. Confused about drug classes and indications.	Some deficiencies. Incomplete understanding of significant side effects and ways to monitor for safety.	Is aware of major medication classes, their indications. Has basic knowledge of management of common side effects.	⊕ Expanded understanding of therapeutic options, drug-drug interactions. Able to select by applying recent information.	⊕⊕ Mastery of drug effects and limits, current with state-of-the-art concepts. Comprehensive understanding of treatment options.
2B. Psychotherapy	Little knowledge beyond the fact that it involves listening and talking.	Marginal concept of types and indications.	Can name the different types of psychotherapy, their indications. Has some concept of background theories and application.	⊕ Familiar with different types of psychotherapies. Good grasp of theories, application, and indications for different types of psychotherapy.	⊕⊕ Excellent grasp of theories, application, and indications of different types of psychotherapy, especially CBT. Understands complex issues and interactions.
2C. Descriptive Psychiatry and Differential Diagnosis	Lacks background knowledge to understand common problems. Cannot interpret data. No prioritization. Likely to miss major disorder. Ignores factors contributing to pathology.	Some difficulty with interpretation of data and prioritization of issues. Sometimes ignores factors contributing to pathology.	Knows major DSM-IV categories and can come up with rational differential diagnoses. Familiar with relevant terminology and can define commonly used descriptive terms.	⊕ Can make DSM-IV and biopsychosocial formulations. Well versed with terminology. Very thorough with differential diagnosis.	⊕⊕ Excellent formulation. Synthesizes detailed differential diagnosis with appropriate prioritization of issues. Expanded grasp of terminology.

3. PRACTICE-BASED LEARNING AND IMPROVEMENT (RESIDENT'S ABILITY TO APPLY DAILY CLINICAL PRACTICE TO OWN LEARNING AND DEVELOPMENT)

	Makes same mistakes again and again. Oblivious of context. No appreciation of ethnic or cultural variations.	Needs frequent prompting to adjust. Slow to learn from previous mistakes. Minimal appreciation of ethnic or cultural variations.	Improves and adds to own development by learning from day-to-day clinical practice. Adapts to cultural backgrounds and work situations without undue assumptions.	⊕ Learns quickly from practice. Anticipates and adapts to different cultural backgrounds and work situations. Assimilates and applies relevant literature.	⊕⊕ Excellent learning from practice. Rapidly acquires, assimilates, and applies relevant literature. Recognizes and utilizes strengths and weaknesses of systems.

4. INTERPERSONAL AND COMMUNICATION SKILLS

4A. Working Relationships	Inappropriate, antagonistic, disruptive, arrogant, not respectful of peers or staff.	Inflexible, inconsiderate, frequently loses composure.	Good team member. Cordial to staff members; recognizes their contributions, knows when to consult others. Invites mutual respect.	⊕ Flexible, supportive, respectful, develops very good rapport with team. Recognizes the benefits and limits of others' skills.	⊕⊕ Poised, establishes tone of mutual respect. Invaluable team member. Recognizes talents within team. Brings out the best in others.
4B. Patient-Specific Skills	Avoids personal contact, tactless, inattentive to patients' feelings, impolite, arrogant, abusive.	Occasionally insensitive or inattentive, superficial. Reluctant to communicate with patients' families.	Empathic, listens attentively, develops rapport, adequate communication with patient and family.	⊕ Effective communication, perceived by patient and family as capable. Can handle some degree of volatility.	⊕⊕ Works directly with patient, inspiring confidence and compliance. Works exceptionally well even with difficult patients.
4C. Verbal Presentation	Inaccurate, major omissions, rambling, inappropriate comments.	Disorganized, unfocused, some omissions. Gives irrelevant or inaccurate information.	Complete, includes all basic information, with positives and relevant negatives. Follows usual format.	⊕ Well organized, thorough, precise. Effectively integrates data. Appreciates subtleties. Concise, comprehensive.	⊕⊕ Polished presentations, tailored to situation. Outstanding, discussion reflects thorough understanding of disorder and patient situation.

5. PROFESSIONALISM

5A. Management of Clinical Responsibility	Is often absent or late. Leaves patient care tasks unfinished. Lacks follow-up. Fails to plan. Misses changes in patient status. Delegates tasks inappropriately to reduce workload. Avoids assigned duty area. Fails to respond to paging. ◯	Occasionally absent or late. Unavailable at times. Sometimes has others do what is assigned to resident. Erratic in planning and follow-up. Slow to see changes in patient status. Unreliable response to paging. ◯	Satisfactory attendance, generally on time. Usually available when needed. Delegates appropriately. Adequate management plans and follow-up. Timely recognition of changes. Reliable response to paging. ◯	⊕ Commendable attendance and punctuality. Always answers pages quickly. Thoughtful, detailed management plans. Regular follow-up, quick to see changes. ◯	⊕⊕ Impeccably punctual, unswervingly diligent, immediately responsive. Anticipates needs. Seeks involvement in all parts of patient care and research. Eager for new skills. Insightful plans and follow-up. Suggests alternative. ◯
5B. Documentation	Inaccurate data. Overdue. Misleading. Disorganized. Important portions missing. Rationale unclear. Change or progress unclear. Copied and pasted without editing. Typos abound. Poor grammar. Poses legal risk. ◯	Occasional inaccuracies, poor organization, but rationale can be deciphered. Moderate risk potential. ◯	Records generally coherent, timely, illustrate progression of treatment, include basic elements to satisfy billing, legal, and future patient care needs. ◯	⊕ Notes timely, clearly show treatment rationale and progress, useful for reference. Medical record appreciated and handled as an integral part of patient care, risk management, and financial accountability. ◯	⊕⊕ Well organized, focused, comprehensive. Records fully recognized as an important part of patient care and as a legal document. Always done completely and promptly, including dictation requirements. ◯
5C. Teaching	Makes no effort to convey information to students and poorly models seeking of information. ◯	Answers students' question briefly if asked, but does not initiate any teaching. ◯	Makes satisfactory effort to instruct and encourage students assigned. Recognizes good teaching opportunities. ◯	⊕ Consistently acknowledged as a teacher by students and other learners. ◯	⊕⊕ Viewed by students and staff as *the* source of clinical and scientific data. Inspires learning and independent research. ◯
5D. Ethical Decision Making, Honesty, Cultural Sensitivity	Does not apply acceptable moral standards to decision making. Often prejudiced. Attempts to camouflage errors. Does not share credit or accept blame. ◯	Irregularly applies acceptable moral standards to decision making. Not always impartial. On occasion covers up mistakes and tends to take more credit than due. ◯	Usually applies acceptable moral standards to personal and clinical decision making. Admits to errors. Generally able to give and take credit appropriately. ◯	⊕ Quality decision making. Always applies sound moral standards to decision making. Admits to errors. Acknowledges equality of all people. ◯	⊕⊕ Exceptional decision making, based on impeccable moral standards. Respects human dignity, without bias. Recognizes responsibility to patient and to society. ◯
5E. Personal Qualities	Does not seek information. Unreliable. Dawdles. Poor initiative. Leaves early and is inflexible. Overestimates ability. Unresponsive to criticism. Frequently looks sloppy. ◯	Inefficient. Requires reminders to seek information. Often unwilling to do what is needed. Fails to seek supervision. Semiresponsive to criticism. Looks untidy at times. ◯	Reads what is essential. Reliable follow-through. Effective time use. Works required time and generally flexible, responsive to criticism. Seeks help when needed. Appears tidy and composed. ◯	⊕ Eager to learn, seeks additional reading. Efficient, conscientious, and helpful. Seeks and responds to feedback. Clear view of limitations. Maintains a professional appearance. ◯	⊕⊕ Highly motivated to expand knowledge and enhance productivity. Goes out of the way to help. Peers ask for advice. Maximizes personal strengths. Looks commendably professional. ◯

6. SYSTEMS-BASED CARE (ABILITY TO ADAPT TO MENTAL HEALTH CARE FUNDING AND TO DIFFERENT TYPES OF DELIVERY SYSTEM)

	Lacks background knowledge to understand common patient problems. Unable to work with electronic records. Patient care plan insupportable. Oblivious to treatment algorithms. ◯	Understands a few common patient problems. Limited ability to work with electronic records. Patient care plan often insupportable. Marginally aware of treatment algorithms. ◯	Cognizant of local patient population trends. Able to tailor patient care to resources available in system. Competent with relevant information technology. Aware of local treatment algorithms. ◯	⊕ Up-to-date with local patient population trends. Well aware of resources. Skillfully tailors patient care. Proficient with relevant information technology. Comfortable with local treatment algorithms. ◯	⊕⊕ Fully aware of local patient trends, available resources. Mastery of information technology. Conforms to and improves upon consensus treatment algorithms. ◯

Overall Rating	Not competent ○	Falls below expectations ○	Good, solid work ○	⊕ Exceeds expectations ○	⊕⊕ Far exceeds expectations ○

Assessment Methods (Select all that apply)	Direct observation ○	Records review ○	Discussion with resident ○	Videotape ○	Other_____ ○

General comments:

Other areas of special talent:

Other areas where more work is needed (please elaborate on all *unsatisfactory* ratings [to the left of the gray column] and any significant discrepancies between overall rating and specific ratings):

I have reviewed this performance evaluation with the resident. _____ Date: _____
                                                                                    (Faculty Signature)
I have reviewed this evaluation with the faculty member. _____ Date: _____
                                                                                    (Resident Signature)

PLEASE RETURN TO LINDA ANDREWS, M.D., VIA INTER-INSTITUTIONAL MAIL BY _____

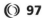

Date reviewed by Residency Director: _____

PGY-III Clinical **Midpoint Feedback** and **Final End of Rotation Evaluation**

Resident's name: _____   Evaluator(s) (please print): _____
Rotation dates: ___/___/200__ to ___/___/200__   Rotation location: _____

A. Midpoint Feedback

Midpoint feedback provided on _____ _____ _____
Date   *Faculty Signature(s)*   *Resident Signature*

B. Final End of Rotation Evaluation

Instructions for scoring: Rate the resident's skill in each of the categories 1–6 using the descriptions as a guide.
Darken bubbles ● with pen or pencil completely. Place emphasis on written comments at the end.

Please note: The gray column identifies competence at satisfactory levels. The two columns to its left denote unsatisfactory performance. The column to the immediate right of the gray column, identified with the symbol ⊕, denotes performance beyond satisfactory levels and is inclusive of the elements specified in the gray column. The extreme right column, identified with the symbol ⊕⊕, includes the *two* elements to its immediate left as well.

1. PATIENT CARE (THE APPLICATION OF KNOWLEDGE IN THE CLINICAL SETTING)

1A. Diagnostic Skills, Assessment, and Evaluation	Unable to summarize and organize psychiatric history. Often rambling or confused.	Disorganized or unfocused. Limited differential diagnosis with some omissions. Lacks biopsychosocial format.	Accurate, comprehensive history with description of intrapsychic and situational conflicts. Careful and complete differential diagnosis.	⊕ Well organized. Able to present coherent and relevant biopsychosocial formulation. A skillful diagnostician.	⊕⊕ Outstanding discussion that reflects thorough understanding of disease and patient situation. Recognizes the value and limitations of various diagnostic tools.
	○	○	○	○	○
1B. Ability to Develop Rapport and Therapeutic Alliance	Frequently unable to engage patient in an interview. Tactless. Disrespectful.	Adversarial with patients. Does not form a therapeutic alliance.	Makes patients comfortable and engages them in the process of evaluation and treatment. Good patient compliance and follow-up.	⊕ Can engage patients well. Perceived as capable. Very respectful. Able to elicit cooperation even in awkward situations.	⊕⊕ Has patient's full confidence. Works exceptionally well even with difficult patients. Maximizes adherence to treatment.
	○	○	○	○	○
1C. Psychotherapy	Unable to establish therapeutic alliance or to formulate treatment plan or goals. Cannot utilize even the most rudimentary strategies of therapy.	Significant deficiencies, but aware of the influence of past experiences on current symptoms. Unable to utilize psychotherapy along with medication.	Appreciates transference, identifies major dynamic themes. Applies appropriate psychotherapeutic techniques, even in the medication management setting. Uses psychotherapeutic skills within clinic setting.	⊕ Comfortable therapist who identifies, understands, and utilizes transference and countertransference. Identifies symptoms more amenable to specific psychotherapeutic technique.	⊕⊕ Actively and aggressively pursues experience in various psychotherapies. Able to incorporate multiple patients into their routine. Manages powerful feelings with grace and efficacy.
	○	○	○	○	○
1D. Pharmacotherapy	Unable to formulate effective drug treatment plans. May be reckless or even dangerous at times.	Usually able to select a first-line treatment. Some understanding of side-effect profiles and symptom focused therapy.	Selects the best drug treatment based on patient's illness, side effects, and drug interactions. Able to appreciate the influence of medical history.	⊕ Algorithmic approach to medication management. Expanded knowledge of options. Able to adapt fund of knowledge to real-world patient situations.	⊕⊕ Outstanding ability to formulate treatment plan that addresses idiosyncracies, refractory cases, and complications. Skilled at maximizing compliance.
	○	○	○	○	○
1E. Treatment Planning	Unreliable. Fails to plan. Misses changes in patient's mental status and/or fails to follow up.	Erratic in planning and follow-up. Slow to see changes in patient status. Does not schedule follow-up visits within appropriate time frames.	Adequate management plans and follow-up with recognition of changes in condition. Appropriate follow-up of patients, sees unstable patients for frequent visits until stable.	⊕ Thoughtful, detailed management. Quickly recognizes changes. Skilled treatment plans in outpatient setting. Avoids unnecessary hospitalization.	⊕⊕ Efficient and insightful management plans with many options and awareness of the risk/benefit of each.
	○	○	○	○	○

1. PATIENT CARE *(continued)*

1F. Patient Communication and Education	No effort to involve patient or to provide information/education. Avoids interaction with patient.	Provides partial information. Little concern for patient autonomy and informed decision making.	Discusses treatment options thoroughly. Actively informs patient of options, risks, etc. Verifies patient understanding of indications of medications, dosing, and side effects.	⊕ Helps patient to feel informed and involved in treatment decisions. Spends extra time to ensure adequate understanding.	⊕⊕ Gains patient's full confidence by carefully explaining complex treatment strategies and empathically establishing a mutual information exchange.
	○	○	○	○	○

2. CLINICAL SCIENCE (FUND OF KNOWLEDGE, INCLUDING CONCEPTUAL THEORY AND SCIENTIFIC LITERATURE)

2A. Pharmacotherapy	Major deficiencies in the fundamentals. No appreciation of advanced techniques. Requires constant and extensive supervision.	Has difficulty applying basic knowledge. Rarely uses secondary or tertiary strategies.	Good fundamental psychopharmacologist who is generally able to apply advanced techniques in difficult and refractory cases.	⊕ Very solid basics. Often suggests alternative strategies and is aware of recent advances in the field. Understands rational approach to combination and augmentation of medications.	⊕⊕ Mastery of fundamental psychopharmacology. Excellent grasp of advanced techniques and in-depth knowledge of the most recent literature.
	○	○	○		○
2B. Psychotherapy	Does not grasp the styles and applications of different types of psychotherapy. Rarely suggests this intervention.	Some difficulty with necessary concepts such as transference, resistance, and defense. Limited appreciation of combined therapy.	Good basic knowledge of various psychotherapies, their unique vocabularies, and applications. Rarely hesitates to employ this treatment.	⊕ Expanded understanding of different strategies, including their complexities and subtleties. Thoughtful about risks and potential benefits of intervention.	⊕⊕ Excellent theoretical psychiatrist who is fluent in the terminology and rationale for various methods. Adept biopsychosocial modeling. Well read in classic and modern literature.
	○	○	○	○	○
2C. Descriptive Psychiatry and Differential Diagnosis	Cannot interpret or synthesize data. No prioritization. Likely to miss major disorder.	Some difficulty with interpretation of data and prioritization of issues.	Forms adequate differential diagnosis with appropriate prioritization of issues.	⊕ Effectively integrates data. Incorporates subtleties. Thoughtful prioritization.	⊕⊕ Understands complex issues and problem interactions.
	○	○	○	○	○

3. PRACTICE-BASED LEARNING AND IMPROVEMENT (RESIDENT'S ABILITY TO APPLY DAILY CLINICAL PRACTICE TO OWN LEARNING AND DEVELOPMENT)

	Unable to incorporate his or her own experience. Limited or no ability to use rounds or patient care as learning experiences.	Struggles to benefit from ward teaching. Erratic response to feedback from faculty and ancillary personnel.	Uses clinical examples to learn treatment planning, differential diagnoses, and follow-up. Steadily adds individual patient data to fund of knowledge.	⊕ Formulates treatment in response to expanded awareness of his or her experience. Uses rating scales and objective measures of efficacy.	⊕⊕ Consistently and accurately utilizes clinical experience to improve patient care. Readily gathers and applies current literature to his or her own patients.
	○	○	○	○	○

4. INTERPERSONAL AND COMMUNICATION SKILLS

4A. Working Relationships	Inappropriately antagonistic, disruptive, arrogant. Dismissive toward staff members.	Inflexible, inconsiderate, frequently loses composure.	Cooperative. Adjusts to circumstances. Valuable team member.	⊕ Flexible, supportive, fosters good rapport within team. Interacts easily with other disciplines.	⊕⊕ Poised, establishes mutual respect with other disciplines. Seen as helpful.
	○	○	○	○	○
4B. Patient-Specific Skills	Avoids contact, tactless, inattentive to patient's feelings.	Occasionally insensitive or thoughtless. May be superficial or callous.	Empathic and attuned. Listens and conveys information easily and effectively.	⊕ Excellent communicator perceived by patient as open, helpful and capable.	⊕⊕ Attains patient's full confidence. Able to work adeptly with even difficult patients.
	○	○	○	○	○

5. PROFESSIONALISM

5A. **Management of Clinical Responsibility**	Inappropriate, antagonistic attitude. Late to clinical responsibilities with no regard to inconvenience of others. Unprepared. Often absent or unreachable.	Usually present but frequently disinterested. Rarely adequately prepared. Cannot keep up with clinical data. Difficult to track down.	Adequately prepared and organized for clinical and educational activities. Delegates appropriately. Solid attendance and availability.	⊕ Ably manages all patient responsibilities and educational experiences. Adept at managing many, complicated patients. Impeccable attendance.	⊕⊕ Superbly organized clinician with exceptional attitude and unusual ability to coordinate care for many, complicated patients while participating fully in educational requirements of residency training.
	○	○	○	○	○
5B. **Documentation**	Inaccurate. Major omissions. Disorganized. No appreciation of the legal risks inherent in charting. Repeated errors in documentation of services and deficiencies in chart reviews.	Unfocused notes with many omissions or marked overinclusion. Many late and/or untimely entries. Records insufficient for documentation of service.	Complete documentation that includes all basic information and satisfies legal expectations. Some awareness of documentation requirements for outpatient reimbursement.	⊕ Well organized and thorough. Precise charting that reflects appreciation for the medical record as a part of patient's care. Documentation necessary for various CPT codes routinely considered.	⊕⊕ Concise without losing completeness. Always timely. Medical record used as an important tool in both patient care, medicolegal affairs, and documentation of services provided.
	○	○	○	○	○
5C. **Teaching**	Never teaches. Often ignores the students or only expects them to provide service.	Rarely teaches and is ineffective when an attempt is made. No active organization of educational endeavors.	Solid clinical teacher who adds didactic sessions to the student's and lower-level resident's workday.	⊕ Above-average bedside teacher who conveys difficult aspects of psychiatric knowledge to learners of all levels.	⊕⊕ Exceptional and enthusiastic teacher. Systematically covers many areas of psychiatry for all members of the team. Regularly arranges educational experiences.
	○	○	○	○	○
5D. **Ethical Decision Making, Honesty, Cultural Sensitivity**	Does not accept moral standards for decision making. Prejudiced. Dishonest. Attempts to cover up errors.	Irregularly applies moral standards. Not always impartial. May try to minimize or camouflage mistakes and shortcomings.	Applies moral standards to personal and clinical decisions relevant to the role of resident. Admits errors. Aware of cultural differences.	⊕ Ethical and reasoned decision making process. Acknowledges equality of all people.	⊕⊕ Exceptional decision-maker who respects human dignity without bias. Utilizes cultural differences to maximize care delivery.
	○	○	○	○	○
5E. **Personal Qualities**	Unreliable and unfocused. No initiative. Inflexible. Takes credit without shouldering blame. Unprofessional in dress and demeanor.	Inefficient. Requires frequent input to motivate. Poorly responsive to feedback. Occasionally inappropriately dressed. Overestimates ability.	Effective and reliable. Flexible person who implements feedback effectively. Appropriately seeks help. Professional appearance and demeanor.	⊕ Eager learner who is efficient, conscientious, and helpful. Seeks feedback. Accepts the inevitability of errors.	⊕⊕ Highly motivated and exceptionally productive. Always helpful. Appropriately seeks new responsibility. Accentuates the abilities of the rest of the team. Shares success and credit readily.
	○	○	○	○	○

6. SYSTEMS-BASED CARE (ABILITY TO ADAPT TO MENTAL HEALTH CARE FUNDING AND TO DIFFERENT TYPES OF DELIVERY SYSTEM)

	No appreciation of the various structures used to provide mental health care. Frequently mismanages patients because of these deficiencies.	Significant weaknesses in ability to adapt treatment to the available resources of patient.	Recognizes the realities of various public and private sector mental health systems. Organizes treatment with regard to payer specifications. Understands algorithms used in public, outpatient settings.	⊕ Thoughtful, detailed management of patients with appropriate regard to patients' financial ability to comply with treatment. Actively seeks additional resources for patients.	⊕⊕ Well versed in current mental health financing including carve-outs, public funding, and private resources. Develops elegant and imaginative strategies to maximize care.
	○	○	○	○	○

Overall Rating	Not competent	Falls below expectations	Good, solid work	⊕ Exceeds expectations	⊕⊕ Far exceeds expectations
	○	○	○	○	○

Assessment Methods (Select <u>all</u> that apply)	Direct observation	Records review	Discussion with resident	Videotape	Other_____
	○	○	○	○	○

General comments:

Other areas of special talent:

Other areas where more work is needed (please elaborate on all *unsatisfactory* ratings [to the left of the gray column] and any significant discrepancies between overall rating and specific ratings):

I have reviewed this performance evaluation with the resident. _____ Date: _____
(Faculty Signature)

I have reviewed this evaluation with the faculty member. _____ Date: _____
(Resident Signature)

PLEASE RETURN TO LINDA ANDREWS, M.D., VIA INTER-INSTITUTIONAL MAIL BY _____

Date reviewed by Residency Director: _____

PGY-IV Clinical **Midpoint Feedback** and **Final End of Rotation Evaluation**

Resident's name: _____ Evaluator(s) (please print): _____

Rotation dates: ___/___/200__ to ___/___/200__ Rotation location: _____

A. Midpoint Feedback

Midpoint feedback provided on _____ _____ _____
                                 Date   *Faculty Signature(s)*   *Resident Signature*

B. Final End of Rotation Evaluation

Instructions for scoring: Rate the resident's skill in each of the categories 1-6 using the descriptions as a guide.
Darken bubbles ● with pen or pencil completely. Place emphasis on written comments at the end.

Please note: The gray column identifies competence at satisfactory levels. The two columns to its left denote unsatisfactory performance. The column to the immediate right of the gray column, identified with the symbol ⊕, denotes performance beyond satisfactory levels and is inclusive of the elements specified in the gray column. The extreme right column, identified with the symbol ⊕⊕, includes the *two* elements to its immediate left as well.

1. **PATIENT CARE** (THE APPLICATION OF KNOWLEDGE IN THE CLINICAL SETTING)

1A. Diagnostic Skills, Assessment and Evaluation	Unable to summarize and organize psychiatric history. Often rambling or confused.	Disorganized or unfocused. Limited differential diagnosis with some omissions. Lacks biopsychosocial format.	Accurate, comprehensive history with description of intrapsychic and situational conflicts. Careful and complete differential diagnosis.	⊕ Well organized. Able to present coherent and relevant biopsychosocial formulation. A skillful diagnostician.	⊕⊕ Outstanding discussion that reflects thorough understanding of disease and patient situation. Recognizes the value and limitations of various diagnostic tools.
	○	○	○	○	○
1B. Ability to Develop Rapport and Therapeutic Alliance	Frequently unable to engage patient in an interview. Tactless. Disrespectful.	Adversarial with patients. Does not form a therapeutic alliance.	Makes patients comfortable and engages them in the process of evaluation and treatment. Good patient compliance and follow-up.	⊕ Can engage patients well. Perceived as capable. Very respectful. Able to elicit cooperation even in awkward situations.	⊕⊕ Has patient's full confidence. Works exceptionally well even with difficult patients. Maximizes adherence to treatment.
	○	○	○	○	○
1C. Psychotherapy	Unable to establish therapeutic alliance or to formulate treatment plan or goals. Cannot utilize even the most rudimentary strategies of therapy.	Significant deficiencies, but aware of the influence of past experiences on current symptoms. Unable to utilize psychotherapy along with medication.	Appreciates transference, identifies major dynamic themes. Applies appropriate psychotherapeutic techniques, even in the medication management setting. Uses psychotherapeutic skills within clinic setting.	⊕ Comfortable therapist who identifies, understands, and utilizes transference and countertransference. Identifies symptoms more amenable to specific psychotherapeutic technique.	⊕⊕ Actively and aggressively pursues experience in various psychotherapies. Able to incorporate multiple patients into their routine. Manages powerful feelings with grace and efficacy.
	○	○	○	○	○
1D. Pharmacotherapy	Unable to formulate effective drug treatment plans. May be reckless or even dangerous at times.	Usually able to select a first-line treatment. Some understanding of side-effect profiles and symptom focused therapy.	Selects the best drug treatment based on patient's illness, side effects, and drug interactions. Able to appreciate the influence of medical history.	⊕ Algorithmic approach to medication management. Expanded knowledge of options. Able to adapt fund of knowledge to real-world patient situations.	⊕⊕ Outstanding ability to formulate treatment plan that addresses idiosyncracies, refractory cases, and complications. Skilled at maximizing compliance.
	○	○	○	○	○
1E. Treatment Planning	Unreliable. Fails to plan. Misses changes in patient's mental status and/or fails to follow up.	Erratic in planning and follow-up. Slow to see changes in patient status. Does not schedule follow-up visits within appropriate time frames.	Adequate management plans and follow-up with recognition of changes in condition. Appropriate follow-up of patients, sees unstable patients for frequent visits until stable.	⊕ Thoughtful, detailed management. Quickly recognizes changes. Skilled treatment plans in outpatient setting. Avoids unnecessary hospitalization.	⊕⊕ Efficient and insightful management plans with many options and awareness of the risk/benefit of each.
	○	○	○	○	○

1. PATIENT CARE (continued)

1F. Patient Communication and Education	No effort to involve patient or to provide information/education. Avoids interaction with patient.	Provides partial information. Little concern for patient autonomy and informed decision making.	Discusses treatment options thoroughly. Actively informs patient of options, risks, etc. Verifies patient understanding of indications of medications, dosing, and side effects.	⊕ Helps patient to feel informed and involved in treatment decisions. Spends extra time to ensure adequate understanding.	⊕⊕ Gains patient's full confidence by carefully explaining complex treatment strategies and empathically establishing a mutual information exchange.
	○	○	○	○	○

2. CLINICAL SCIENCE (FUND OF KNOWLEDGE, INCLUDING CONCEPTUAL THEORY AND SCIENTIFIC LITERATURE)

2A. Pharmacotherapy	Major deficiencies in the fundamentals. No appreciation of advanced techniques. Requires constant and extensive supervision.	Has difficulty applying basic knowledge. Rarely uses secondary or tertiary strategies.	Good fundamental psychopharmacologist who is generally able to apply advanced techniques in difficult and refractory cases.	⊕ Very solid basics. Often suggests alternative strategies and is aware of recent advances in the field. Understands rational approach to combination and augmentation of medications.	⊕⊕ Mastery of fundamental psychopharmacology. Excellent grasp of advanced techniques and in-depth knowledge of the most recent literature.
	○	○	○	○	○
2B. Psychotherapy	Does not grasp the styles and applications of different types of psychotherapy. Rarely suggests this intervention.	Some difficulty with necessary concepts such as transference, resistance, and defense. Limited appreciation of combined therapy.	Good basic knowledge of various psychotherapies, their unique vocabularies, and applications. Rarely hesitates to employ this treatment.	⊕ Expanded understanding of different strategies, including their complexities and subtleties. Thoughtful about risks and potential benefits of intervention.	⊕⊕ Excellent theoretical psychiatrist who is fluent in the terminology and rationale for various methods. Adept biopsychosocial modeling. Well read in classic and modern literature.
	○	○	○	○	○
2C. Descriptive Psychiatry and Differential Diagnosis	Cannot interpret or synthesize data. No prioritization. Likely to miss major disorder.	Some difficulty with interpretation of data and prioritization of issues.	Forms adequate differential diagnosis with appropriate prioritization of issues.	⊕ Effectively integrates data. Incorporates subtleties. Thoughtful prioritization.	⊕⊕ Understands complex issues and problem interactions.
	○	○	○	○	○

3. PRACTICE-BASED LEARNING AND IMPROVEMENT (RESIDENT'S ABILITY TO APPLY DAILY CLINICAL PRACTICE TO OWN LEARNING AND DEVELOPMENT)

	Unable to incorporate his or her own experience. Limited or no ability to use rounds or patient care as learning experiences.	Struggles to benefit from ward teaching. Erratic response to feedback from faculty and ancillary personnel.	Uses clinical examples to learn treatment planning, differential diagnoses, and follow-up. Steadily adds individual patient data to fund of knowledge.	⊕ Formulates treatment in response to expanded awareness of his or her experience. Uses rating scales and objective measures of efficacy.	⊕⊕ Consistently and accurately utilizes clinical experience to improve patient care. Readily gathers and applies current literature to his or her own patients.
	○	○	○	○	○

4. INTERPERSONAL AND COMMUNICATION SKILLS

4A. Working Relationships	Inappropriately antagonistic, disruptive, arrogant. Dismissive toward staff members.	Inflexible, inconsiderate, frequently loses composure.	Cooperative. Adjusts to circumstances. Valuable team member.	⊕ Flexible, supportive, fosters good rapport within team. Interacts easily with other disciplines.	⊕⊕ Poised, establishes mutual respect with other disciplines. Seen as helpful.
	○	○	○	○	○
4B. Patient-Specific Skills	Avoids contact, tactless, inattentive to patient's feelings.	Occasionally insensitive or thoughtless. May be superficial or callous.	Empathic and attuned. Listens and conveys information easily and effectively.	⊕ Excellent communicator perceived by patient as open, helpful and capable.	⊕⊕ Attains patient's full confidence. Able to work adeptly with even difficult patients.
	○	○	○	○	○

5. PROFESSIONALISM

5A. Management of Clinical Responsibility	Inappropriate, antagonistic attitude. Late to clinical responsibilities with no regard to inconvenience of others. Unprepared. Often absent or unreachable.	Usually present but frequently disinterested. Rarely adequately prepared. Cannot keep up with clinical data. Difficult to track down.	Adequately prepared and organized for clinical and educational activities. Delegates appropriately. Solid attendance and availability.	⊕ Ably manages all patient responsibilities and educational experiences. Adept at managing many, complicated patients. Impeccable attendance.	⊕⊕ Superbly organized clinician with exceptional attitude and unusual ability to coordinate care for many, complicated patients while participating fully in educational requirements of residency training.
	○	○	○	○	○
5B. Documentation	Inaccurate. Major omissions. Disorganized. No appreciation of the legal risks inherent in charting. Repeated errors in documentation of services and deficiencies in chart reviews.	Unfocused notes with many omissions or marked overinclusion. Many late and/or untimely entries. Records insufficient for documentation of service.	Complete documentation that includes all basic information and satisfies legal expectations. Some awareness of documentation requirements for outpatient reimbursement.	⊕ Well organized and thorough. Precise charting that reflects appreciation for the medical record as a part of patient's care. Documentation necessary for various CPT codes routinely considered.	⊕⊕ Concise without losing completeness. Always timely. Medical record used as an important tool in both patient care, medicolegal affairs, and documentation of services provided.
	○	○	○	○	○
5C. Teaching	Never teaches. Often ignores the students or only expects them to provide service.	Rarely teaches and is ineffective when an attempt is made. No active organization of educational endeavors.	Solid clinical teacher who adds didactic sessions to the student's and lower-level resident's workday.	⊕ Above-average bedside teacher who conveys difficult aspects of psychiatric knowledge to learners of all levels.	⊕⊕ Exceptional and enthusiastic teacher. Systematically covers many areas of psychiatry for all members of the team. Regularly arranges educational experiences.
	○	○	○	○	○
5D. Ethical Decision Making, Honesty, Cultural Sensitivity	Does not accept moral standards for decision making. Prejudiced. Dishonest. Attempts to cover up errors.	Irregularly applies moral standards. Not always impartial. May try to minimize or camouflage mistakes and shortcomings.	Applies moral standards to personal and clinical decisions relevant to the role of resident. Admits errors. Aware of cultural differences.	⊕ Ethical and reasoned decision making process. Acknowledges equality of all people.	⊕⊕ Exceptional decision-maker who respects human dignity without bias. Utilizes cultural differences to maximize care delivery.
	○	○	○	○	○
5E. Personal Qualities	Unreliable and unfocused. No initiative. Inflexible. Takes credit without shouldering blame. Unprofessional in dress and demeanor.	Inefficient. Requires frequent input to motivate. Poorly responsive to feedback. Occasionally inappropriately dressed. Overestimates ability.	Effective and reliable. Flexible person who implements feedback effectively. Appropriately seeks help. Professional appearance and demeanor.	⊕ Eager learner who is efficient, conscientious, and helpful. Seeks feedback. Accepts the inevitability of errors.	⊕⊕ Highly motivated and exceptionally productive. Always helpful. Appropriately seeks new responsibility. Accentuates the abilities of the rest of the team. Shares success and credit readily.
	○	○	○	○	○
5F. Administrative Skills	Unable to supervise or inappropriately supervises. Cannot make decisions. Fails to complete paperwork and reports.	Marginally effective at supervision. Inconsistent appreciation for necessary documentation standards and paperwork.	Able to coordinate and supervise a team. Good planner. Ensures that necessary documentation is complete and timely.	⊕ Easily adapts to the administrative and supervisory role. Independently coordinates team function.	⊕⊕ Exemplary organizer, supervisor, leader. Fosters excellence within team. Encourages compliance with documentation and required paperwork.
	○	○	○	○	○

6. SYSTEMS-BASED CARE (ABILITY TO ADAPT TO MENTAL HEALTH CARE FUNDING AND TO DIFFERENT TYPES OF DELIVERY SYSTEM)

	No appreciation of the various structures used to provide mental health care. Frequently mismanages patients because of these deficiencies.	Significant weaknesses in ability to adapt treatment to the available resources of patient.	Recognizes the realities of various public and private sector mental health systems. Organizes treatment with regard to payer specifications. Understands algorithms used in public, outpatient settings.	⊕ Thoughtful, detailed management of patients with appropriate regard to patients' financial ability to comply with treatment. Actively seeks additional resources for patients.	⊕⊕ Well versed in current mental health financing including carve-outs, public funding, and private resources. Develops elegant and imaginative strategies to maximize care.
	○	○	○	○	○

Overall Rating	Not competent	Falls below expectations	Good, solid work	⊕ Exceeds expectations	⊕⊕ Far exceeds expectations
	◯	◯	◯	◯	◯

Assessment Methods (Select all that apply)	Direct observation	Records review	Discussion with resident	Videotape	Other_____
	◯	◯	◯	◯	◯

General comments:

Other areas of special talent:

Other areas where more work is needed (please elaborate on all *unsatisfactory* ratings [to the left of the gray column] and any significant discrepancies between overall rating and specific ratings):

I have reviewed this performance evaluation with the resident. _____ Date: _____
(Faculty Signature)

I have reviewed this evaluation with the faculty member. _____ Date: _____
(Resident Signature)

PLEASE RETURN TO LINDA ANDREWS, M.D., VIA INTER-INSTITUTIONAL MAIL BY _____

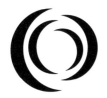

Psychotherapy Supervision Evaluation

PSYCHOTHERAPY SUPERVISION EVALUATION

PGY-II, -III, and -IV

Please provide formal, midpoint feedback and complete the signature blanks below *quarterly* during the psychotherapy supervision period.

Please complete the entire evaluation form semiannually (usually December and June) during the supervision period.

Resident: _____ Supervisor: _____

Dates of evaluation: _____

Quarterly review (verbal feedback) provided on _____ . Resident: _____

Supervisor: _____

Information source (check all that apply): Resident report Direct observation Videotape
Audiotape Record review Other _____

Instructions: *Using the key below, please indicate level of competency by circling the appropriate number 1–5. If the category is not appropriate to PGY level or therapeutic experience, please circle N/A.*

1 Not competent	2 Approaching competency	3 Satisfactorily competent	4 Highly competent	5 Exceptionally competent	N/A Not applicable

I.   FUNDAMENTAL PSYCHOTHERAPY SKILLS

IA. Boundaries

1. Ability to manage therapeutic boundaries, including personal space, handling of gifts, confidentiality, etc.	1 2 3 4 5
2. Ability to define therapeutic contract with patient, including time, fee setting, and collections	1 2 3 4 5

IB. Therapeutic Alliance

1. Ability to establish rapport and form a therapeutic alliance	1 2 3 4 5
2. Ability to interact nonjudgmentally and empathically	1 2 3 4 5
3. Ability to recognize cultural/religious influence in therapeutic process	1 2 3 4 5

IC. Resistance/Defenses

1. Ability to recognize resistances and deal with them effectively to maintain stability of the therapeutic process	1 2 3 4 5
2. Ability to recognize and use transference and countertransference in the therapeutic process	1 2 3 4 5

ID. Goals

1. Understands the indications and contraindications for the major therapeutic modalities (dynamic, CBT, IPT)	1 2 3 4 5
2. Selects an appropriate therapy model for a specific patient	1 2 3 4 5
3. Assesses the patient's progress in therapy	1 2 3 4 5
4. Manages the termination phase effectively	1 2 3 4 5

1 Not competent	2 Approaching competency	3 Satisfactorily competent	4 Highly competent	5 Exceptionally competent	N/A Not applicable

II.   SUPPORTIVE PSYCHOTHERAPY

1.	Ability to identify defense mechanisms while supporting adaptive defenses	1	2	3	4	5	N/A
2.	Ability to assume an active stance including ego lending and ego building	1	2	3	4	5	N/A
3.	Ability to elicit and appropriately contain affect	1	2	3	4	5	N/A
4.	Ability to employ crisis intervention techniques	1	2	3	4	5	N/A
5.	Ability to utilize stress management techniques	1	2	3	4	5	N/A

III.   PSYCHODYNAMIC PSYCHOTHERAPY

1.	Ability to recognize central dynamic issues	1	2	3	4	5	N/A
2.	Ability to conceptualize a psychodynamic formulation	1	2	3	4	5	N/A
3.	Ability to link understanding of the patient's past, present, and transference patterns to thoughts, feelings, and behaviors	1	2	3	4	5	N/A
4.	Ability to describe patient's major defensive organization	1	2	3	4	5	N/A
5.	Ability to clarify, confront, and make interpretations at appropriate times	1	2	3	4	5	N/A

IV.   COMBINED PSYCHOTHERAPY AND PSYCHOPHARMACOLOGY

1.	Ability to integrate psychotherapeutic and psychopharmacologic interventions in a mutually beneficial manner so that neither is neglected	1	2	3	4	5	N/A
2.	Ability to conduct a complete medication assessment within the context of a psychotherapeutic process, while making interpretations and empathic comments	1	2	3	4	5	N/A
3.	Ability to appreciate the potential psychodynamic issues around the prescribing of medications (resistance, compliance, transitional object, etc.)	1	2	3	4	5	N/A
4.	Ability to assess suicidality on an ongoing basis as it relates to the prescribing of potentially dangerous medications	1	2	3	4	5	N/A
5.	Ability to provide education about medications in a manner that complements the psychotherapeutic technique, appreciating the limitations of each treatment modality	1	2	3	4	5	N/A

1 Not competent	2 Approaching competency	3 Satisfactorily competent	4 Highly competent	5 Exceptionally competent	N/A Not applicable

V.   COGNITIVE BEHAVIORAL PSYCHOTHERAPY

1. Ability to set a collaborative agenda for each session, manage time limits, and foster the patient's eventual termination and self-management   1   2   3   4   5   N/A

2. Ability to help the patient recognize automatic thoughts, maladaptive assumptions, and core beliefs/schemas   1   2   3   4   5   N/A

3. Ability to identify and alter cognitive distortions in order to alleviate symptoms   1   2   3   4   5   N/A

4. Ability to help patients develop new, more rational responses to automatic thoughts and core beliefs   1   2   3   4   5   N/A

5. Ability to design and help patients plan and implement behavioral experiments, such as activity monitoring with reward paradigms, in vivo exposure, and relaxation   1   2   3   4   5   N/A

VI.   BRIEF PSYCHOTHERAPY

1. Ability to recognize a patient with sufficient ego strength and psychological mindedness to pursue brief psychotherapy   1   2   3   4   5   N/A

2. Familiarity with the many models and paradigms used in brief psychotherapy, including supportive techniques, dynamic/expressive options, and manualized techniques   1   2   3   4   5   N/A

3. Awareness that central to all brief psychotherapies is the concept of focus, not global characterological change   1   2   3   4   5   N/A

4. Ability to work in the markedly accelerated models of time-limited therapy while still maintaining a therapeutic alliance and holding environment   1   2   3   4   5   N/A

5. Ability to work toward effective termination from the outset of treatment   1   2   3   4   5   N/A

COMMENTS:

<u>Semiannual review</u>   DATE: _____

SIGNATURE: _____ SIGNATURE: _____

                Resident   Supervisor

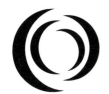

Verification of Resident's Experience Tracking Form

Verification of Resident's Experience

Resident name: _____

Date entered BCM Residency Program: _____

_____ Months of primary care (internal medicine, pediatrics, or family practice) (**4 months** minimum)

_____ Months of neurology (1 of the **2 months** minimum may be in child neurology)

_____ Months of adult inpatient psychiatry (**9 months** adult inpatient minimum; 18 months maximum)

_____ Months of continuous adult outpatient psychiatry (**12 FTE months** minimum)

_____ Months of child and adolescent psychiatry (**2 months** minimum, not required if resident is completing training in child and adolescent psychiatry)

_____ Months of consultation-liaison (**2 months** minimum with adults)

_____ **1 month** of geriatric psychiatry

_____ **1 month** of addiction psychiatry

_____ Elective rotations

He/she has had experience in: (please check)

_____ Emergency psychiatry   _____ Forensic psychiatry
_____ Psychotherapy   _____ Continuity experience with psychotic patients
_____ Community psychiatry   _____ Continuity experience with nonpsychotic patients

Dates of semiannual evaluation: _____

Dates of review of cognitive exam: _____

Dates of review of practical exam (Mock Boards): _____

Dates of review of patient log documentation: _____

Date left BCM Residency Program: _____

Date completed BCM Residency Program: _____

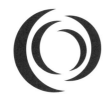

Semiannual Evaluation Summary Form

Semiannual Evaluation Summary Form

Resident name:

PGY:

Semiannual evaluation date:

Six months covered by this semiannual evaluation:

Clinical assignments during 6-month evaluation period:

1.

2.

3.

General summary of written evaluations:

Log card documentation:

Seminar and journal club attendance:

PRITE or Mock Board performance:

Awards or honors received during this reporting period:

1.

2.

Areas of particular strength/skill:

1.

2.

Areas requiring attention/improvement:

1.

2.

Suggestions/goals for professional growth/
  achievement:

1.

2.

_____
Linda B. Andrews, M.D.
Director of Residency Education

_____
John W. Burruss, M.D.
Associate Director of Residency Education

Resident feedback:

_____
Resident signature

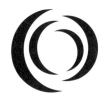

Verification of Resident's Achieved Competency Form

Verification of Resident's Achieved Competency

Resident name: _____ PGY: _____

Date entered BCM Residency Program: _____ Semiannual evaluation date: _____

Date completed BCM Residency Program: _____

Competency measured	Assessment method(s)	Yes	No	Competence achieved (date)
General Competencies				
Patient Care	Clinical evaluations			
Medical Knowledge	PRITE scores Clinical evaluations			
Practice-Based Learning and Improvement	Journal club presentations Clinical evaluations			
Interpersonal and Communication Skills	Psychotherapy evaluations Mock Board examination Interviewing seminar videotape Empathy seminar videotape Case conference presentation(s) Clinical evaluations			
Professionalism	Medical student teaching feedback Psychotherapy evaluations Chief resident evaluation Clinical evaluations			
Systems-Based Practice	Clinical evaluations			
Psychotherapy Competencies				
Brief Therapy	Psychotherapy evaluations Clinical evaluations			
Cognitive-Behavioral Therapy	Psychotherapy evaluations Clinical evaluations			
Combined Psychotherapy and Psychopharmacology	Psychotherapy evaluations Mock Board examination Clinical evaluations			
Psychodynamic Therapy	Psychotherapy evaluations Empathy seminar videotape Mock Board examination Case conference presentation(s) Clinical evaluations			
Supportive Therapy	Psychotherapy evaluations Interviewing seminar videotape Mock Board examination Clinical evaluations			

This verification form should be completed as part of the midyear semiannual evaluation for each PGY-II, -III, and -IV resident. A resident will be reported as "Competence Achieved" for his/her level of training in a given competency area once he/she receives six positive (yes) measures of competence without any negative (no) measures indicating a failure to achieve competence.

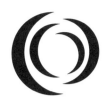

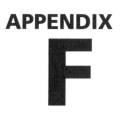

Evaluation Method Summary Forms by Postgraduate Year

Evaluation Methods PGY-I

Evaluation type	Evaluation frequency	Competencies assessed
Clinical rotation faculty written evaluation (includes daily direct observation of resident) (global rating, checklist, record review)	Monthly (12 total)	All 6 General Competencies Supportive Psychotherapy
Multiple-choice question (MCQ) examination	Once per year	Medical Knowledge
Videotaped patient interview (peer review; part of 360-degree global rating)	Once per year	Patient Care Interpersonal and Communication Skills Professionalism
Nursing written evaluation (part of 360-degree global rating)	Monthly at HCHD (6 total)	Interpersonal and Communication Skills Professionalism
Patient experience logs (case logs)	Logs reviewed twice per year	Patient Care Medical Knowledge
Chart review (record review)	Daily at HCHD for 6 months	Patient Care Medical Knowledge Interpersonal and Communication Skills Professionalism Systems-Based Practice
Seminar evaluation (12 seminars)	Each seminar evaluated once per year (12 total)	All 6 General Competencies
Program director semiannual evaluation (in-person review of all written evaluations) (global rating)	Twice per year	All 6 General Competencies
Progressions Committee meetings (peer review)	Monthly (12 total)	All 6 General Competencies
Outcomes Curriculum (checklist, peer review)	Quarterly meetings (4 meetings per year)	All 6 General Competencies
Ethics Curriculum (Introduction to Forensics/Ethics)	8 sessions (seminar)	Professionalism Practice-Based Learning and Improvement Systems-Based Practice
Research Curriculum (Introduction to Evidence-Based Psychiatry)	4 sessions (seminar)	Practice-Based Learning and Improvement

Evaluation Methods PGY-II

Evaluation type	Evaluation frequency	Competencies assessed
Clinical rotation faculty written evaluation (includes daily direct observation of resident) (global rating, checklist, record review)	Monthly (12 total)	All 6 General Competencies
Multiple-choice question (MCQ) examination	Once per year	Medical Knowledge
Videotaped patient interview (peer review; part of 360-degree global rating)	Once per year, as part of 18-session empathy seminar	Patient Care Interpersonal and Communication Skills Professionalism Psychodynamic Psychotherapy
Patient experience logs (case logs)	Logs reviewed twice per year	Patient Care Medical Knowledge
Chart review (at VAMC) (record review)	Daily at VAMC for 2–4 months	Patient Care Medical Knowledge Interpersonal and Communication Skills Professionalism Systems-Based Practice
Psychotherapy supervision written evaluations (2 supervisors) (global rating, record review)	Twice per year (4 evaluations total)	Patient Care Medical Knowledge Interpersonal and Communication Skills Professionalism All 5 Psychotherapy Competencies
Mock Board examination (OSCE)	Once per year	All 6 General Competencies
Seminar evaluation (25 seminars)	Each seminar evaluated once per year (25 total)	All 6 General Competencies Psychodynamic Psychotherapy Cognitive Behavioral Therapy Combined Psychotherapy and Psychopharmacology
Journal club presentation evaluation (checklist)	Once per year	Medical Knowledge Interpersonal and Communication Skills Practice-Based Learning and Improvement Systems-Based Practice
Program director semiannual evaluation (in-person review of all written evaluations) (global rating)	Twice per year	All 6 General Competencies
Progressions Committee meetings	Monthly (12 total)	All 6 General Competencies All 5 Psychotherapy Competencies
Outcomes Curriculum (checklist, peer review)	Quarterly meetings (4 meetings per year)	All 6 General Competencies
Ethics Curriculum (Advanced Ethics)	4 sessions	Professionalism Practice-Based Learning and Improvement Systems-Based Practice
Research Curriculum (Essentials of Evidence-Based Psychiatry)	8 sessions (seminar)	Practice-Based Learning and Improvement
Cultural Psychiatry seminar	5 sessions	Professionalism
Quality Assurance seminar	12 sessions	Practice-Based Learning and Improvement Systems-Based Practice

Evaluation Methods PGY-III

Evaluation type	Evaluation frequency	Competencies assessed
Clinical rotation faculty written evaluation (includes daily direct observation of resident) (global rating, checklist, record review)	Twice per year (rotation assignments 6 months each)	All 6 General Competencies All 5 Psychotherapy Competencies
Multiple-choice question (MCQ) examination	Once per year	Medical Knowledge
Nursing written evaluation (part of 360-degree global rating)	Twice per year	Interpersonal and Communication Skills Professionalism
Patient experience logs (case logs)	Logs reviewed twice per year	Patient Care Medical Knowledge
Chart review (all rotations) (record review)	Daily at all rotation assignments	Patient Care Medical Knowledge Interpersonal and Communication Skills Professionalism Systems-Based Practice
Psychotherapy supervision written evaluations (2 supervisors) (global rating, record review)	Twice per year (4 evaluations total)	Patient Care Medical Knowledge Interpersonal and Communication Skills Professionalism All 5 Psychotherapy Competencies
Mock Board examination (OSCE)	Once per year	All 6 General Competencies All 5 Psychotherapy Competencies
Seminar evaluation (15 seminars)	Each seminar evaluated once per year (15 total)	All 6 General Competencies All 5 Psychotherapy Competencies
Journal club presentation evaluation (checklist)	Once per year	Medical Knowledge Interpersonal and Communication Skills Practice-Based Learning and Improvement Systems-Based Practice
Program director semiannual evaluations (in-person review of all written evaluations) (global rating)	Twice per year	All 6 General Competencies All 5 Psychotherapy Competencies
Progressions Committee meetings (peer review)	Monthly (12 total)	All 6 General Competencies All 5 Psychotherapy Competencies
Outcomes Curriculum (checklist, peer review)	Quarterly (4 per year)	All 6 General Competencies
Ethics Curriculum (Advanced Ethics)	10 sessions (seminar)	Professionalism Practice-Based Learning and Improvement Systems-Based Practice
Research Curriculum (Advanced Evidence-Based Psychiatry)	5 sessions (seminar)	Practice-Based Learning and Improvement
Teaching Residents to Teach seminar	4 sessions	Professionalism Interpersonal and Communication Skills Practice-Based Learning and Improvement
Leadership seminar	7 sessions	Professionalism Systems-Based Practice

Evaluation Methods PGY-IV

Evaluation type	Evaluation frequency	Competencies assessed
Clinical rotation faculty written evaluation (includes daily direct observation of resident) (global rating, checklist, record review)	4 times per year (rotation assignments usually 3 months each)	All 6 General Competencies All 5 Psychotherapy Competencies
Multiple-choice question (MCQ) examination	Once per year	Medical Knowledge
Patient experience logs (case logs)	Logs reviewed twice per year	Patient Care Medical Knowledge
Chart review (at Baylor Psychiatry Clinic [BPC]) (record review)	Twice per year (at BPC)	Patient Care Medical Knowledge Interpersonal and Communication Skills Professionalism Systems-Based Practice
Psychotherapy supervision written evaluation (2 supervisors) (global rating, record review)	Twice per year (4 evaluations total)	Patient Care Medical Knowledge Interpersonal and Communication Skills Professionalism All 5 Psychotherapy Competencies
Mock Board examination (OSCE)	Once per year	All 6 General Competencies All 5 Psychotherapy Competencies
Seminar evaluation (9 seminars)	Each seminar evaluated once per year (9 total)	All 6 General Competencies All 5 Psychotherapy Competencies
Program director semiannual evaluation (in-person review of all written evaluations) (global rating)	Twice per year	All 6 General Competencies All 5 Psychotherapy Competencies
Progressions Committee meetings	Monthly (12 total)	All 6 General Competencies All 5 Psychotherapy Competencies
Transition to Practice seminar	9 sessions	Professionalism Practice-Based Learning and Improvement Systems-Based Practice
Leadership seminar	7 sessions	Professionalism Systems-Based Practice
Administrative Psychiatry rotation	3–6 months (each resident)	All 6 General Competencies

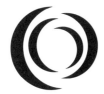

Completion of Training Letter

Completion of Training
  Letter: _____

_____ began his/her training in general psychiatry at Baylor College of Medicine on _____ and is expected to complete his/her training on _____. _____ generally met (or exceeded or far exceeded) expectations for residents at his/her level of training on all categories of evaluation. He/she demonstrated particular interest in _____. He/she performed _____ on the PRITE and on exams of clinical competence.

He/she will have completed the following time-based general psychiatry required rotations:

____ months internal medicine
____ months neurology
____ months pediatrics
____ months adult inpatient psychiatry
____ months continuous outpatient psychiatry
____ months child and adolescent psychiatry
____ months consultation-liaison psychiatry
____ months geriatric psychiatry
____ months addiction psychiatry

  He/she will also have met program requirements in forensic psychiatry, community psychiatry, neuropsychiatry, emergency psychiatry, psychotherapy, continuity of experience with psychotic patients, and continuity of experience with nonpsychotic patients. _____ performed in an ethical manner and related satisfactorily with colleagues. _____ had no documented evidence of unethical or unprofessional behavior in his/her training record. At the time of graduation, he/she demonstrated sufficient professional ability to practice competently and independently.

_____   _____

Linda B. Andrews, M.D.   Date
Director of Residency Education

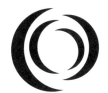

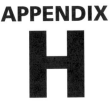

Example Goals and Objectives for Didactic Courses and Rotations

The authors acknowledge and thank Dr. Joseph D. Hamilton for his participation in creating the items in this appendix.

EXAMPLE COURSE GOALS AND OBJECTIVES

Teaching Residents to Teach

Coordinators: Linda Andrews, M.D., and J.D. Hamilton, M.D.

Introduction

This seminar will meet for four sessions, as shown on the **schedule** below. Syllabus materials are attached. If you wish to purchase a **textbook,** we would recommend *The Physician as Teacher* (2nd edition), by Thomas L. Schwenk and Neal Whitman. However, it is a bit costly, and some chapters from it are photocopied as part of the syllabus material.

The objectives of the seminar are that you should

1. Recognize that most medical encounters are opportunities to teach (patients, families, students, residents, colleagues). **Practice-Based Learning**
2. Understand the aims and methods of teaching in several different settings (large group, small group, bedside/rounds). **Systems-Based Practice**
3. Learn how to give feedback to medical students or other trainees. **Practice-Based Learning, Interpersonal and Communication Skills**
4. Become aware of the strengths and weaknesses of your own teaching style.
5. Recognize anticipated teaching dilemmas you will encounter next year as administrative chief residents, and develop possible solutions for them.
6. Learn skills to help make teaching enjoyable.

The **format** of the seminar will be four 1¼-hour sessions with leaders discussing specific material and demonstrating (in collaboration with you) the points and techniques discussed. Our goal is for the sessions to be interactive and practical.

The **evaluation** of your performance in the seminar will be based upon the following:

1. **Attendance**—We expect you to attend every seminar session unless you're ill, on vacation (or other authorized absence), or in the middle of an emergency. Please inform Dr. Andrews' office if you plan to be absent.
2. **Participation**—We expect you to participate in the interactive exercises and to discuss your own experiences and concerns about teaching.

We will also be seeking an evaluation from you about the seminar and its session leaders.

Schedule for Fall 2003

All sessions are on **Tuesdays, 8:15–9:30** A.M., **in Room 728.**

Date	Session Leader	Topic
September 24	J. Burruss, M.D.	Bedside/rounds teaching
October 1	V. Hamilton, M.D.	Giving feedback
October 8	L. Andrews, M.D.	Small group teaching
October 15	R. Pesikoff, M.D.	Large group teaching

Introduction

This seminar on Descriptive Psychiatry will be meeting weekly for the next several months. A detailed schedule is enclosed, along with the syllabus materials.

The **text** for the seminar is *Diagnostic and Statistical Manual of Mental Disorders*, 4th Edition, Text Revision (the large version, not the pocket one), known familiarly as DSM-IV-TR, which is available in the Baylor bookstore. We recommend that you buy the hardcover version, because the paperback won't stand up well to repeated use and is almost as overpriced.

The **objectives** of the seminar are that, by the end of the seminar, you should

- Appreciate the usefulness and limitations of the descriptive viewpoint in psychiatric diagnosis.
- Understand the basic assumptions and concepts of descriptive psychiatry.
- Know standardized definitions of common signs and symptoms of psychopathology and reliably recognize such signs and symptoms.
- Be familiar with the classification and criteria of mental disorders in DSM-IV-TR system and in alternative descriptive schemes covered in the seminar.
- Be able to make reliable descriptive psychiatric diagnoses using DSM-IV-TR criteria.

As the objectives indicate, the seminar primarily concerns diagnosis and usually will not address etiology or treatment. The information in this course is generally applicable to the "Medical Knowledge" general competency of the ACGME.

The **format** of each session, after two general ones, will be to cover a group of mental disorders, sometimes along with a related group of symptoms of psychopathology. For each such session, you'll be assigned to read (ahead of time) the syllabus outline, the relevant sections in DSM-IV-TR, and sometimes journal articles. You'll also be given a "case of the week" case report on which to practice DSM-IV-TR diagnosis and to discuss the differences and ambiguities we discover. For the first case of the week (in session 1), the seminar leaders will discuss the diagnosis and diagnostic reasoning as a demonstration. Each week thereafter, one of you will be assigned to formally present how you arrived at your diagnosis for the case of the week; as part of this presentation, you'll construct and distribute a timeline of the significant symptoms in the case. After this presentation, the rest of the group will discuss how their diagnoses agree or differ. Assignments for the initial presentation of the case of the week are listed on the session schedule. You're free to exchange these assignments, but everyone should be prepared to discuss the case of the week every week. If the assigned person is unavailable for any reason, we'll call on someone else to begin discussion of the case. In addition, we'll sometimes view and discuss short portions of videotaped patient interviews from a descriptive diagnostic standpoint. Other than the case of the week and the videotapes, the content of each session will be determined by your own questions and discussion about the session topics.

The **evaluation** of your seminar performance will be based on the following criteria:

- *Attendance*—We expect you to attend every seminar session except when you're ill, on vacation, on an authorized absence, or in the middle of an emergency. Please notify Dr. Hamilton or Dr. Garza if you're going to be absent.
- *Participation*—We expect your discussion in the seminar to show appropriate progress toward reaching the objectives listed above. We particularly value questions and comments that show a critical analysis of the seminar material and a willingness to express independent opinions.

We'll give you an informal midcourse evaluation (for your eyes only) about midway through the seminar, and a cumulative evaluation (to be shared with Dr. Andrews) at the end of the seminar. At those same times, we'll also ask you to evaluate the seminar sessions and our performance as seminar leaders.

EXAMPLE ROTATION GOALS AND OBJECTIVES

Ben Taub Inpatient Service and Ben Taub Psychiatric Emergency Unit

FIRST POSTGRADUATE YEAR
LIST OF ROTATIONS

Ben Taub Inpatient Service
Ben Taub Psychiatric Emergency Unit

KEY for General Competencies indicated for all goals and objectives

Patient Care **PC**
Medical Knowledge **MK**
Interpersonal and Communication Skills **ICS**
Practice-Based Learning and Improvement **PBL**
Professionalism **P**
Systems-Based Practice **SBP**

Ben Taub Inpatient Service

1. The resident will participate in the multidisciplinary team for diagnosis and treatment objectives. The resident will be supervised by a staff psychiatrist who will direct the interdisciplinary team. The resident's experience will allow the following:

   A. Development of skills in the psychiatric interview. **(PC, ICS)**
   B. Development of skills in diagnosis and classification. **(PC)**
   C. Development of skills in formulations of problems, objectives of treatment, methods of treatment, and evaluations of treatment. **(PC)**
   D. Development of an appreciation of psychology, social work, and occupational therapy's relationships to psychiatry. **(SBP)**
   E. Development of understanding and using social work reports, group therapy reports, psychological measurements, and occupational therapy reports to assess and treat patients. **(SBP)**

2. The resident under a staff psychiatrist supervisor will participate as the primary physician for up to eight patients. The patient population will be varied and will primarily comprise the organic disorders, schizophrenia, affective disorders, other functional psychoses, neurotic disorders, personality disorders, mental disability, parasuicide, and dependency on alcohol and other drugs. **(PC, MK, P, ICS)**

3. The resident will observe and direct patients in a therapeutic community. **(PC, ICS)**

4. The resident will observe family interviews. They will participate, where indicated, with social work in couples and family therapy of their patients. **(PC, P, ICS)**

5. The resident will develop skills and knowledge in the use of psychotropic drug treatment, as well as ECT and other somatic therapies where indicated. **(PC, MK)**

6. The resident will develop skills and knowledge in individual supportive psychotherapy. **(PC, MK, Supportive Psychotherapy)**

7. The resident will be encouraged to participate as an observer in group therapy of his/her patients. **(PC)**

8. The resident will participate with psychology in developing behavioral treatment interventions when appropriate. **(SBP)**

9. The resident will develop knowledge and skills in evaluation and execution of commitment procedures. **(PC, MK)**

10. The resident will be expected to interface with other medical disciplines in the medical care of his/her patients. **(SBP, ICS)**

11. The resident will participate in the assessment and rehabilitation of short-term patients. He/she will participate in directing follow-up care and social placement of all their patients. **(SBC)**

12. The resident will be encouraged to develop a collegial relationship with fellow residents and staff as well as serve as role models for medical students. **(P, ICS)**

13. The resident will participate with the Multidisciplinary Team in addressing ethical dilemmas in psychiatry. **(P, ICS)**

Ben Taub Psychiatric Emergency Unit (1-South)

Goals

1. To provide PGY-I residents with an appropriate exposure in forensic and emergency psychiatry. **(PC, MK)**
2. To expose PGY-I residents to principles of crisis intervention. **(PC, MK, SBC)**
3. To help PGY-I residents develop a basic knowledge in acute psychopharmacologic interventions. **(MK)**

Objectives

1. To provide basic information concerning involuntary treatment. **(MK)**
2. To develop skills in forensic-related psychiatric issues. **(PC)**
3. To help develop knowledge in the utilization of psychotropic medications in acute psychiatric emergencies. **(PC, MK)**
4. To provide experience in crisis intervention and resolution. **(PC)**
5. To learn the use of antipsychotic agents in rapid tranquilization methods. **(PC, MK)**
6. To learn appropriate clinical assessments of suicide patients. **(PC, MK, ICS)**
7. To learn how to conduct emergency psychiatric evaluations. **(PC, MK)**
8. To learn availability of community resources for referral purposes. **(SBP)**
9. To learn how to differentiate psychiatric emergencies from medical/surgical emergencies in which the prominent presentation involves psychiatric symptoms. **(PC, MK)**
10. To learn how to triage psychiatric patients to the appropriate level of care. **(PC, MK)**

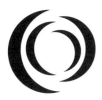

Index

Page numbers in **boldface** *type refer to tables.*

Jay Bahm
802-399-9838